Hank Ratris
11/13/13

✗

The Compatibility Gene

DANIEL M. DAVIS

The Compatibility Gene

How Our Bodies Fight Disease,
Attract Others, and Define Our Selves

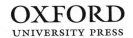

OXFORD

UNIVERSITY PRESS

OXFORD
UNIVERSITY PRESS

Oxford University Press is a department of the University of Oxford.
It furthers the University's objective of excellence in research, scholarship,
and education by publishing worldwide.

Oxford   New York
Auckland   Cape Town   Dar es Salaam   Hong Kong   Karachi
Kuala Lumpur   Madrid   Melbourne   Mexico City   Nairobi
New Delhi   Shanghai   Taipei   Toronto

With offices in
Argentina   Austria   Brazil   Chile   Czech Republic   France   Greece
Guatemala   Hungary   Italy   Japan   Poland   Portugal   Singapore
South Korea   Switzerland   Thailand   Turkey   Ukraine   Vietnam

Oxford is a registered trade mark of Oxford University Press in the UK and certain other countries.

Published in the United States of America by
Oxford University Press
198 Madison Avenue, New York, NY 10016

Library of Congress Cataloging-in-Publication Data
Davis, Daniel M. (Daniel Michael), 1970–
The compatibility gene : how our bodies fight disease, attract others, and define our selves / Daniel M. Davis.
pages cm
Includes bibliographical references and index.
ISBN 978-0-19-931641-0 (hardback)
1. Medical genetics. 2. Infection—Immunological aspects. 3. Immunogenetics. 4. Human molecular genetics. I. Title.
RB155.D36 2014
616'.042—dc23   2013020914

3 5 7 9 8 6 4 2

Printed in the United States of America on acid-free paper

For Katie, Briony and Jack

Contents

Acknowledgements

I am especially grateful to those I had the privilege of interviewing for this book: Brigitte Askonas, Gary Beauchamp, Pamela Bjorkman, Walter Bodmer, Leslie Brent, Derrick Brewerton, Mary Carrington, Margaret Dallman, Mark Davis, Elizabeth Dexter, Peter Doherty, Ron Germain, Klas Kärre, Jim Kaufman, Rolf Kiessling, Steve Marsh, Polly Matzinger, Hugh McDevitt, Andrew McMichael, Charles Medawar, Avrion Mitchison, Ashley Moffett, Jon van Rood, Eric Schadt, Carla Shatz, Elizabeth Simpson, Andrew Strominger, Jack Strominger, Alain Townsend, Bruce Walker, Claus Wedekind, Wayne Yokoyama and Rolf Zinkernagel. Several discussions with Peter Parham were particularly influential.

I also thank Steve Marsh and the team at Anthony Nolan, who performed the HLA typing for my wife and me. Others who helped me to address specific issues while writing this book include Danny Altmann, Jorge Carneiro, Andrew Giddy, Salim Khakoo, Ofer Mandelboim, Jim McCluskey, Maryam Mehrabi, Sophie Pageon, Marco Purbhoo and Anton van der Merwe. I'm also indebted to those who commented on early versions of some or all of the text: Brigitte Askonas, Mary Carrington, George Cohen, Richard Dawkins, Peter Doherty, Steve Marsh, Peter Parham, Elizabeth Simpson, Jack Strominger and Claus Wedekind. Of course, any remaining errors are my responsibility alone.

Many others supported me while writing this book, including members of my research team, the senior faculty at Imperial College London, who allowed me to take a year's sabbatical leave, and faculty at the University of Manchester, where I completed the project. Armand Leroi, author of *Mutants*, was exceptionally helpful throughout, pushing me to develop my ideas more carefully at the outset and showing me where to rework the text at the end. Caroline Hardman, my agent initially at the Christopher Little Literary Agency and now at Hardman and Swainson, has been fantastic throughout and gave useful feedback at every stage. Sarah Levitt at the Zoë Pagnamenta Agency also had an important input in improving my text. Alice Brown, Lucy Hairsine, Clive Gerner and Joel Rickett all helped my proposal get noticed early on.

I'm indebted to Stefan McGrath and William Goodlad at Penguin Press, who supported this project at the outset. My editor at Penguin Press, Thomas Penn, author of *The Winter King*, had a wonderful influence on my writing and the structure of this book. My editor at OUP, Joan Bossert, also made many very helpful, formative suggestions. I'm also grateful to David Watson, who carefully copy-edited my text. Finally, my wife, Katie, edited the book first and suggested many important changes; I thank her, and our kids, Briony and Jack, for encouraging me throughout and sharing the journey.

A Brief Note to Professional Scientists

Immunology is a vast and complex science. In this book, I have sought to present some of the big ideas alongside the stories of individuals who have played a central role in gaining this knowledge. But I am acutely aware that there are a huge number of people who contributed to our understanding of the immune system and the relevant genetics, who are not explicitly named in this book or have been mentioned only superficially. I have made many ruthless omissions in my attempt to keep the narrative and the scientific ideas as clear as possible for the general reader. Quite simply, this is an extraordinarily rich story in which there have been many players, and it's impossible to catalogue everyone's contribution. Immunologists will notice that some details are covered more thoroughly than others; I have discussed class I genes far more than class II genes, for example. Rather than present a complete textbook-level description of the immune system, I wanted to focus on broad issues, such as the variation in human immune-system genes which can, for example, be illustrated equally well with class I or class II genes. I can only apologize to anyone whose discoveries I have not included or have mentioned all too briefly; *any one book can only tell part of a story.*

Introduction

There's a man, happy and minding his own business, who sees an open gate in the corner of the room where he is. He approaches the gate, wondering where it leads. But as he does so, he sees that it's being guarded. The guard – who looks powerful from a distance but appears unkempt close up – warns the man that nobody has ever been through this gate. He also mentions that beyond this gate there's another, with a guard who's even more powerful. So the man just backs away and spends his days – which turn into decades – in the room, occasionally wondering about the gate and where it leads to. Eventually, when the man is weak and knows his own death must be near, he realizes what he should ask the guard. He shuffles back and asks, 'In all the time I've been in this room, why has nobody ever been through the gate?' 'Because,' the guard replies, 'this gate was only meant for you . . . but it's too late now.'

Written in 1914, Franz Kafka's parable 'Before the Law' has inspired me often. The version that I carry in my head now is slightly different from what Kafka actually wrote, or the way Anthony Hopkins tells it in the 1993 movie of *The Trial*. There are many interpretations of any great allegory; this one works for me on two levels. First, as a scientist, I want to open doors to where nobody has been before. Second, there is the simple, but all-too-easy-to-forget, truth that each of us really is unique, right down to the molecular detail of what our bodies are made of. My aim is for this book to work on these two levels. I want to tell some inspiring stories of men and women who have fought their way to new rooms of knowledge and describe how, from the vantage point they reached, we see a fundamental importance for our own personal uniqueness.

Essentially, this is the story of a few human genes and how we discovered what these genes do. The knowledge we now possess of these genes reveals a great beauty in how we work at a microscopic – and macroscopic – level. We are not merely a more-or-less average blend of our parents; rather we gain specific traits and characteristics through the individual genes we inherit. As human beings we each have around 25,000 genes. To a large extent, we each have a very similar set of these genes but there are variations that provide us with individual characteristics such as hair and eye colour. Genetic variation also gives us more subtle – and superficially undetectable – differences. Crucially, the genes in this story are those that vary the *most* from person to person. These genes are, in effect, a molecular mark that distinguishes each of us as individuals.

It is this feature that led to their discovery. These genes – we'll call them our compatibility genes (though their unwieldy formal name is the *major histocompatibility complex* or MHC genes) – are not uniquely human and they were first discovered in mice. During the 1930s, scientists were trying to understand what determines the acceptance or rejection of skin cells transplanted from one mouse to another. They observed that transplanted cells were rejected when they had different compatibility genes; transplantation worked well when these genes were matched. In the 1950s and '60s, this was also found to be true for humans, and today, these are the genes that, when matched between donors and recipients, help provide the best chance of success in many types of organ transplantation. But the normal job for these genes can't be to make life difficult for transplant surgeons. What do these genes really do?

Decades of patient scientific inquiry and the occasional stroke of genius have unravelled the workings of our compatibility genes. This book charts this human endeavour – a global adventure spanning sixty years – tracing the history of transplants and immunology, leading to our eventual understanding of how and why compatibility genes are crucial to our health. This amounts to a scientific revolution, but not one that came from a single eureka moment; rather a revolution in our understanding of the human body that emerged from a swell of ground-breaking ideas and experiments happening in different places across the globe over decades.

We will see that a great many people made vital contributions – and that their characters do not fit any particular mould of scientist. Some collected data while others contributed more theoretically. Many classified and ordered the information, while others explored more like artists. Often one didn't appreciate another's approach. A picture of science emerges in which hundreds of researchers – each digging away in their own experiments and thoughts – individually uncover a fragment of the big picture.

The view we now have of what these few genes do reveals much about how your immune system works; how your body can detect what is not part of you, such as germs or transplanted organs from someone else. That is to say that these few genes help your body distinguish *self* from *non-self*. Practically – as a consequence of the way this system has evolved – we each have a different set of these genes. And it can really matter which versions you have inherited.

Each of our 25,000 genes can be ranked according to which are most important for our susceptibility or resistance to any given disease. The outcome is that compatibility genes come out top in influencing our susceptibility or resistance to an enormous array of illnesses: multiple sclerosis, rheumatoid arthritis, type I diabetes, psoriasis, leprosy, ankylosing spondylitis and many others.[1]

Take one example: In 2003, Doug Robinson, forty-six, from Truro, Massachusetts, was infected with HIV. Yet, ten years on, his immune system has managed to keep it in check: the virus is almost undetectable in Doug's blood.[2] About 1 in 300 people infected with HIV do not progress to full-blown AIDS for seven years or more, because, like Doug, their immune system is able to fight the virus effectively. But what is so special about Doug's immune system that allows him to do this? Why is Doug so, *so* lucky? Doug's super-power turns out to be a version of compatibility gene that he inherited – one that appears to be particularly beneficial in fighting HIV.

For people infected with HIV, their rate of progression to AIDS depends on, amongst other things, which variants of compatibility genes they have inherited. Doug has a version designated as B*57 (said as B-fifty-seven), which happens to be one that protects most effectively against the progression of HIV to AIDS. Protection against disease is surely enough to warrant a book about how these genes work, but in fact, their importance stretches further. There is evidence that these very same genes are linked to whole other areas of human biology.

Radical and provocative research has suggested that finding a lover might be made simpler: as a 'scientific' process in which there's no need to waste time looking in bars or at parties. Just take a swab and run it along your inside cheek. Put it in an envelope and fill out the brief form – not forgetting to include your customer number. Send it off, wait a few days, then log in to your online account. Having analysed your DNA, your ideal partner will be selected from a company's database. Just go ahead and arrange a date. Marriage, happiness and wonderful kids are all assured, with minimal risk of either one of you ever cheating.

This highly controversial view of what's possible is based on experiments that suggest that you find others more or less sexy according to which type of compatibility genes they have. There have even been claims that women experience higher rates of orgasm if they choose partners with the right set of compatibility genes. The experiment that started this line of thinking used a very unusual protocol for scientific work.

Women were to refrain from sex for two days, use a nasal spray to keep their nostrils clear, read Patrick Süskind's novel *Perfume* – a book about a man with olfactory hypersensitivity who is obsessed with people's smells – and then come into the lab to smell a collection of T-shirts worn by men who hadn't showered for two days. The experiment yielded an astonishing result: T-shirts worn by people with *different* compatibility genes smelt the sexiest. The big idea that follows from this research is that we subconsciously favour sexual partners who have different compatibility genes from ourselves. Profoundly personal, life-forming and life-changing decisions can, it appears, be reduced to the actions of a few inherited genes.

Is this true? How and why could it possibly work? We each spend a great deal of effort defining our personalities by choosing the things we like or dislike, and form friendships with people who have similar tastes. Many of us spend a great deal of our lives in the quest for a soul-mate. The idea of genes pervades our culture, and we have no problem accepting that our physical characteristics – hair and eye colour, for example – are dictated by our genetic make-up. But can something that feels as intimate as choosing a partner be similarly influenced by our genetic inheritance? There's no short answer to this question; the subject is contentious.

Controversy surrounding compatibility genes doesn't stop there. Other research suggests these genes might also influence parts of our brain. Specifically, the wiring between some neurons may be kept or broken according to the activity of compatibility genes. Most recently, evidence has emerged to suggest that compatibility genes are also able to influence the chance that two people have a successful pregnancy.

Quite simply, it seems that these few genes can affect who's born and who dies – at many levels. This multi-functionality of compatibility genes suggests that all of these different aspects of us could be fundamentally connected. And if so, then a shocking amount of who we are and what we do is directly influenced by the way we have evolved to survive disease.

Understanding this in depth – resolving the controversies – is not simply a matter of academic interest. Given, for example, that we each respond slightly differently to any particular disease, it can be expected that we also respond slightly differently to any given medicine. In the not-too-distant future, we can anticipate that vaccines or a choice of therapeutic drugs might be tailored to match our compatibility genes. Unlocking the secrets of our compatibility genes is undoubtedly important for medical practice in the twenty-first century.

Other sorts of issues also arise from these discoveries. The possibility is already available to seek a partner according to compatibility genes,[3] and disease treatments tailored to our gene types are just around the corner. But how much of this is where we want to go? Governments and the pharmaceutical industry must move forward mindfully, so that we don't end up in a Brave New World. We must each make our own personal decisions, fully informed about how this wondrous system works within each of us and across us all.

As I mentioned, there are many interpretations of any great allegory. In Kafka's 'Before the Law', the man and guard might be one and the same; there's an internal struggle in anyone stepping forward somewhere new. More importantly, it is surely impossible that a gate will be opened and closed to fit the term of one person's life. More likely, once a new room has been seen, its guard will not actually be able to shut the gate.

PART ONE

The Scientific Revolution in Compatibility

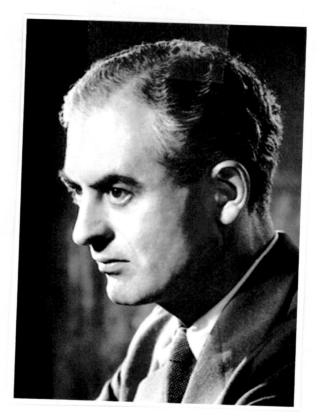

Peter Medawar

I

Frankenstein's Holy Trinity

You can always find stories that make any person look good or bad – with the exception of Peter Medawar. Anecdotes about Medawar always cast him as a hero, and his story is a scientific legend forged from his Nobel-Prize-winning discoveries in transplantation. His work helped reveal how the human body is able to sense its own cells and tissue. Concerned with the difficulties in medical transplantation, he studied how the body is able to accept its own tissue as *self*, yet reacts against alien tissue from somebody else – as *non-self*. His work helped uncover that this happens because a handful of human genes provide a molecular mark of our individuality – 'the uniqueness of the individual', as he called it. These genes are, in effect, hallmarks etched on all our cells which can be recognized by our immune system. Medawar's discoveries are a good place to begin this sixty-year-long scientific adventure to understand how the immune system works, which culminates in recent discoveries indicating that our immune system impacts many aspects of human biology. This journey to understand the importance of our compatibility genes – and Medawar's legend – starts with a plane crash in Oxford in the summer of 1940.

It was a hot Sunday afternoon when Medawar, then twenty-five, enjoying garden life in Oxford with his wife Jean and eldest daughter Caroline, was startled by the sight and noise of a bomber flying low towards them. Jean scrambled with Caroline to a shelter and the plane crashed violently in a garden 200 metres away. It was a British plane and the pilot survived but suffered horrific burns. The sight of such agony marked an epiphany for Medawar: from that moment, his work ceased to be a purely intellectual exercise. 'A scientist who wants to do something original and important must experience, as I did, some kind of shock that forces upon his intention the kind of problem that it should be his duty and will become his pleasure to investigate,' he said later.[1]

Medawar had trained as a zoologist, but his recent research had been to find out which antibiotics were best at treating burns. For the pilot who had just crashed, doctors were at their wits' end in deciding the right medication and asked Medawar to help. They asked him to come and look at the patient, and the visceral shock of pacing the war wounds hospital spurred the young Medawar to think and work to a degree of intensity that he hadn't known he was capable of; Jean said that from then on, 'he worked like a demon'.[2] He saw airmen with much of their skin incinerated, lying in agony: while their lives could be prolonged by new medical advances – blood transfusions and antibiotics – there was no way of treating these horrific burns.

The research that Medawar would carry out in response to this shock marked the beginning of modern transplantation. Even so, it's been said by one of his many protégés, Avrion Mitchison, that his smartest achievement was actually to marry Jean, three years before the formative plane crash.[3] Peter and Jean met as undergraduates in Oxford in 1935, on Peter's twentieth birthday, and they would be married for fifty years, until Peter's death. Physically attractive and charming, Peter was 6 feet 5 inches tall; you 'sensed that you were in the presence of a giant', as one colleague wrote about him.[4] He was vibrant and sharp and had a gift for inspiring those around him. Highly talented, multilingual and also physically attractive herself, Jean was nevertheless in awe of Peter's intellect and charisma.

Peter and Jean's wedding reception was a low-key sherry party in their Oxford flat, the day before Peter's twenty-second birthday. Jean, already twenty-three, had bought her own wedding ring 'to save him time', and their relationship was to remain somewhat unconventional. Once, Jean asked Peter directly if he could spend less time in his lab, to which he replied, 'You have first claim on my love, but not on my time.' Jean thought to argue back – love needs shared time – but she kept quiet. They came to an arrangement in which Peter's time for thinking and working was treasured and protected.[5]

Peter forever remained detached from any emotional problems that might otherwise take up his time and energy, and was generally dismissive of any problems at home. Living frugally during the war years took time and energy and Jean understood this to be her job – leaving Peter to work ferociously. When Peter looked as though he was thinking deeply, Jean would ask 'Are you thinking?' before starting any discussion. If he was, she wouldn't continue.[6] Peter also told Jean that he was happy for theirs to be an open marriage. Peter's discoveries were hard-won, and home life could not have been the bliss it was made out to be in the autobiographies by himself and his wife. He devoted himself fully to solving the transplantation problem.

Skin transplants, or grafts, were needed to treat such extensive burns, but when doctors transplanted skin from one person to the next, it was destroyed two to three weeks later. At the time, doctors didn't think there was any fundamental biological problem to transplantation, only that the actual practicalities had to be perfected; the cutting and sewing. Still, they did know that grafts using skin taken from elsewhere on the same patient worked far better. Why was that? Isn't everybody's skin – human tissue – essentially the same? How could one person's skin differ from that of another? Stranger still, how does your body know the difference?

Medawar's work would help show that transplant rejection is the result of a reaction from immune cells and, crucially, he went on to lead a team that found a way to circumvent transplant incompatibility. In doing so, he went down in scientific history and, aged forty-five, won the Nobel Prize in 1960 for a plethora of crucial experiments. While the medical need for transplantation was made acute by the war, his discoveries answered questions that were not new at all, but ancient.

The basic idea of skin transplantation stretches back for millennia. The renowned Hindu medical text the *Sushruta Samhita* discusses how to extend a short earlobe with skin taken from the patient's cheek or neck.[7] It's not entirely clear where or when Sushruta lived, perhaps between 600 and 400 BCE, and he may have been a contemporary of Buddha. Nor is it clear when this ancient Sanskrit text was written: the version we have now is likely the collective work of many ancient Indian medical practitioners. Nevertheless, this text describes fifteen specific procedures for fixing earlobes, from reconstructing earlobes shortened by a blow, to helping anyone born with short or malformed earlobes who simply wanted enlargements.

Another notable ancient case of transplantation is a third-century CE story of Christian Saints Cosmas and Damian, depicted in a fifteenth-century Spanish iconographic painting held by the Wellcome Trust in London. The most famous miraculous procedure these two early Arabian physicians performed was the replacement of a church official's ulcerated leg with one from a dead Ethiopian. In the painting, their patient is at peace – remarkably so given that his own leg would need to be removed and his new leg attached without anaesthetic. What exactly happened in this early attempt at transplantation is not recorded, but the story is significant for being the first extant description of a concept that was obviously considered even then: that body parts from a dead person might help someone alive.

Nevertheless, it wasn't until four centuries later that transplantation was generally considered a medical possibility – gaining traction from the nineteenth-century view of the human body being machine-like to some extent, with the implication that its parts might be changed or replaced. Indeed, one of the most powerful and pervasive images of dead body parts being used in someone living comes in Mary Shelley's *Frankenstein*. Its publication, on New Year's Day 1818, marked the birth of science fiction as we would recognize it now, and it triggered a fertile debate between art and science that remains vibrant two centuries later.[8] In Shelley's novel, the scientist Victor Frankenstein is obsessed with chemistry and its transformative power. He creates a life from dead body parts but is repulsed by his nameless creation, which in turn becomes lonely and monstrous.

A source of inspiration for Shelley's *Frankenstein* was real-life scientist Humphry Davy.[9] Davy, President of the Royal Society 1820–27, had isolated many substances for the first time, including sodium and calcium, and invented the miner's safety lamp (his protégé Michael Faraday was the father of electricity). Davy advocated that life worked through basic chemistry; that is, living things follow just the same physical and chemical principles as everything not alive. Whether or not you consider that something of us exists beyond chemistry and physics, the immediate implication of Davy's writing, back in the early nineteenth century, was that mankind could use basic chemistry and physics to interrogate and intervene with living things. This thesis was, of course, central to Mary Shelley's narrative – and this way of thinking was essential for the consideration of transplantation as a real possibility.

The cutting and sewing was also crucial and, in 1902, a twenty-nine-year-old French scientist, Alexis Carrel, demonstrated the possibility of stitching blood vessels together (for which he would win the Nobel Prize ten years later). Yet, at the outbreak of the Second World War, there remained a seemingly insurmountable barrier to the use of transplantation for burns victims: the human body could only accept grafts of its own skin and not one from anyone else. Solving this problem required an understanding of why it was that the body should be able to discriminate itself from all other living selves.

So how can scientists approach understanding this – even at a glance, the problem is formidable. How did the scientist who led the way for us solving the problem of transplantation – Medawar – begin? First he needed to study the issue carefully and systematically, and for this he thought it would be useful to immerse himself in a burns unit – to be surrounded by the problem he so wanted to do something about. He obtained a grant from the War Wounds Committee of the UK's Medical Research Council and left home to spend two months in a low-star hotel to work in the Burns Unit of the Glasgow Royal Infirmary, where patients and facilities for research were both available. He was assigned to work with Scottish surgeon Tom Gibson – intelligent and good-looking, Medawar said of him later – and the two became good friends. Together, they set out to observe in minute detail exactly what happened during the process of graft rejection.

Their first patient was a twenty-two-year-old woman, named in papers only as 'Mrs McK'. She had been rushed to the Glasgow Royal Infirmary with deep burns down her right side from falling against her gas fire.[10] The burns were cleaned and a month later she had a blood transfusion but she remained poorly, her wounds still not healed. If her condition had been better, Medawar and Gibson would have grafted large pieces of her own skin to cover the wound, but they decided instead to try several small squares of skin, with the hope that these would grow to cover the whole burnt area. One area of her wound was covered with fifty-two small discs of skin from her thigh and another area with fifty discs of skin taken from her brother's thigh.

Over the following days, the two sets of grafts were studied and biopsies taken for closer examination under a microscope. At first, both grafts looked identical: this was significant as it showed that initially each graft healed properly. But then, a few days later, the microscope revealed that Mrs McK's immune cells had invaded the skin grafts taken from her brother. Between fifteen and twenty-three days after the transplant, the brother's grafts degenerated: Mrs McK's body had rejected them. Her immune cells had seemingly caused the graft rejection, but the evidence was weak: the immune cells were at the scene – but did they do the killing? Medawar and Gibson knew all too well that there were several theories as to what caused transplant rejection and that they would need more than just this circumstantial evidence.

Crucially, Gibson happened to mention to Medawar his suspicion that, in his experience, a second set of skin grafts often degenerated even faster. Medawar recognized this faster reaction second time around as the hallmark of an immune response, and so together they realized that they should systematically test whether or not Gibson's impression was true. To do this, they decided that a second set of discs of her brother's skin should be grafted on Mrs McK. This time, the brother's skin degenerated in about half the time the first skin grafts had lasted. It seemed to bear out Gibson's hunch and was strong evidence that the grafts were rejected because of a reaction involving cells from Mrs McK's immune system. With that, the surgery of transplantation became linked with a scientific realm that was more respectable at the time – understanding the immune system.

Although this was a pivotal observation, it came from only one patient. Medawar knew that an experiment with one patient couldn't be counted as definitive proof of any general principle; he needed large amounts of data – and to get this, he needed to use animals. Back in Oxford, Medawar chose the rabbit – 'more for its size and ease of supply than for any intrinsic merit', he explained to the War Wounds Committee.[11] Taking twenty-five rabbits, he grafted pieces of skin from each one onto every other rabbit in the group. For so many grafts between rabbits, he devised his own methods that are basically still used today – published across two very long papers in 1944 and 1945[12] – and he then stained, examined and photographed hundreds of rabbit-skin samples under the microscope. He also cared for the rabbits himself, looking after their food and their cages and carrying them back and forth for the experiments. If you've ever wondered what it might take to win a Nobel Prize, this one starts here: with an important hypothesis tested by 625 operations on 25 rabbits (25 × 25 individual skin grafts).

The experiments were tough – the hardest work of his life, Medawar later recalled. Sometimes he didn't get home until 11.30 p.m., with a briefcase full of papers to read by morning;[13] he exhausted himself but was spurred on by the thought that it was the least he could do for those actually fighting the war. Medawar was also motivated by ideas: fundamental ideas about the way the world worked and the way that we work. Unlike some great scientists – Einstein, for example, who famously used 'thought experiments' or *Gedankenexperiments* – Medawar's ideas came to him when pondering his experimental results rather than by thinking about abstract concepts alone. Even much later, when he became the head of the UK's National Institute of Medical Research (working in a building used as the fictitious psychiatric hospital Arkham Asylum in the 2005 movie *Batman Begins*), Medawar always sustained his data-driven perspective, setting aside two weekdays and Saturday morning for doing experiments, and never allowing the demands of policy and administration to dominate him.

The outcome of Medawar's meticulous work in the early–mid-1940s was confirmation that skin could not be permanently grafted from genetically different rabbits; as with the grafts from Mrs McK's brother, they lasted a few weeks at best. His experiments also revealed that, in a second round of grafts, rejection happened more quickly. Again, this was exactly what he and Tom Gibson had observed in the Glasgow Infirmary with Mrs McK: the signature of an immune cell response. But, tinkering with the conditions of the rabbit experiments, Medawar now made two other key observations.

First, larger skin grafts were destroyed more rapidly than smaller ones. This feels counter-intuitive: it might be expected that a larger skin graft would simply take longer to be destroyed, given that there's more of it to get rid of. Yet the fact that a larger skin graft was actually destroyed more rapidly indicates an immune response because immune cells would be expected to mount an attack in proportion to the level of threat. A larger graft would, in this view, be attacked more ferociously and destroyed more quickly.

Most importantly, however, Medawar also found that the rate of rejection second time around depended on the relationship between the two grafts. That is, if the second skin graft was taken from a different rabbit from the first, it would be rejected slowly. Only if the second skin graft was from the same donor rabbit as the first would the recipient's body recognize it, having been seen before, and consequently destroy it rapidly. The rabbit's immune system, in other words, had programmed itself to eliminate a particular rabbit's skin, not just any skin graft. It's the same idea when you recover from flu: you'll be strong at fighting the same flu again, but not a different version of flu or some other virus.

Medawar's 625 rabbit operations together amounted to unequivocal evidence that graft rejection was caused by a reaction from the recipient's immune cells. From then on, the thrust of his science was centred on obtaining an intimate understanding of this process of immune rejection – and looking for ways to circumvent it, in order to allow transplantation from anyone to anyone. He never switched to become immersed in studying the human immune system in general – understanding infections, for example; the focus was always on transplantation, the problem he had to solve.[14]

The rabbit experiments, however, were just the prelude to Medawar's most glorious discoveries. In 1947, Medawar – by then aged thirty-two – took up a position of Professor of Zoology at Birmingham University. There, and continuing in University College London, where he moved to in 1951, he led a series of profound experiments, culminating in three and a half pages in the journal *Nature* in 1953,[15] the same year that Watson and Crick famously published the iconic double helix structure of DNA. Today, a new scientific paper is published every thirty minutes, and the vast majority of these papers have little impact beyond the industry of research science. Only very rarely does something sublime appear: something of either exceptional medical importance or something that changes the way we understand ourselves. These three and a half pages could claim to be both.

In these few pages Medawar established a way to solve the problem of transplantation. That is, he found a way to transplant skin from one animal to another so that it would not be rejected – there would be no immune reaction at all – even if the animals were unrelated. The way in which he solved the problem built upon an observation made many years earlier. In science, in general, bolts from the blue can occur – like the discovery of radioactivity by Marie and Pierre Curie and Henri Becquerel in the late 1890s – but these are exceptionally rare. Even with radioactivity, understanding the initial observation certainly didn't come in a flash of inspiration but required a long, hard slog. In Medawar's case, the important foundation for his seminal three and a half pages in 1953 was a paper published eight years earlier by Ray Owen at Wisconsin University in the US.[16] Owen's work was initially ignored by most, and indeed Medawar was unaware of it until he read a paper published in 1949, by Australians Macfarlane Burnet and Frank Fenner, which quoted Owen's research.

Owen discovered that the blood of non-identical cattle twins contained cells in common, presumably coming from the shared placenta. It would be easy to dismiss this as just vaguely interesting; an anecdote of anatomy. But in the context of transplantation, the observation was startling because it meant that each twin of a non-identical pair would not react adversely to cells from the other, even though they were genetically different. The importance of Owen's finding was that this showed that it was at least possible for cells from one animal to exist in another without any reaction occurring: the holy grail for solving the transplantation problem. Inspired, Medawar set out to try to artificially recreate this natural situation in the lab, and this put him on the right track for solving the transplantation problem, and producing his three-and-a-half-page masterpiece.

Medawar worked on the project with his two research team-mates Rupert 'Bill' Billingham and Leslie Brent, who both moved with him from Birmingham to University College London in 1951. Billingham and Brent are far less renowned today than Medawar is; all three investigators played a pivotal role, but Medawar was their undisputed leader. Medawar arrived in London three months before

Billingham and Brent to prepare the three large newly renovated laboratory rooms that they would move into.

Brent was the youngest of the three, aged twenty-six, and the research would form part of his PhD thesis. He had impressed Medawar while working with him as an undergraduate student. Brent's story is one of amazing achievement after an early life of adversity. He was born Lothar Baruch in Köslin, Germany, in 1925 to Jewish parents who were not wealthy but comfortable. His mother wanted him to become a cantor, leading the synagogue congregation in prayer.[17] However, by the time he was eleven, things had become intensely difficult.

Later in life, Brent vividly recalled hiding behind a curtain in his parents' home as a march went past the house and hearing people singing: 'And when Jewish blood spurts from the knife then all is really well.'[18] The men who were marching belonged to the notorious Sturmabteilung, also known as brownshirts, after the paramilitary uniforms they wore, and it was an anti-Semitic lyric they frequently sang, years before the Holocaust.[19] This was the Nazi group who, later in 1938, would be responsible for coordinated attacks on thousands of Jewish shops on *Kristallnacht*. One of Brent's teachers at school was a member of the Sturmabteilung and sometimes taught in full uniform.[20] It bothered him that the only Jew in the class was one of his best pupils. In one instance Brent was made to stand in front of his class while his teacher gave a Nazi diatribe.

Thankfully, Brent's parents knew the director of a Jewish boys' orphanage in Berlin, Kurt Crohn, who had left Köslin when young. One day, in the winter of 1936, Brent went by train to the orphanage, where it turned out that many Jewish boys – even those with parents – had been sent under similar circumstances.

However, the orphanage would offer only a temporary sanctuary. In 1938 it was ransacked by a mob while the thirteen-year-old Brent hid under the roof rafters with a friend. 'There we stayed with beating hearts,' he later recalled, 'until everything became eerily quiet.'[21] Shortly after, on 1 December 1938, a few weeks after *Kristallnacht*, his life was saved by being transported to England, in the Refugee Children's Movement, or *Kindertransport*, programme. Crohn, the orphanage head, had nominated him to be one of the first to travel. Brent remembers how, when they reached Holland, en route to England, they finally 'seemed to have been relieved of [their] role as scapegoats, villains and victims'.[22] Many other boys in the orphanage were not so lucky: they were later rounded up and sent to concentration camps. Crohn himself was killed in Auschwitz in September 1944.

At Dovercourt Reception Camp in Essex – a Butlin's seaside holiday camp used as temporary accommodation for refugee children in 1938–9 – Brent was introduced to English culture and, appearing on a BBC TV documentary aimed at encouraging British couples to take in these new immigrant children, he said he wanted to become a cook. Transferred to a boarding school, he spent his holidays with various families, and, when he was sixteen, a secretary of the Refugee Children's Movement found him a job as a laboratory assistant at Birmingham University. Army service followed. He was in the British infantry from January 1944 to autumn 1947, and it was during this time that he chose his name to be Leslie Brent – Leslie after the actor Leslie Howard and Brent just chosen from telephone directory to have the same initials as the name his parents gave him. He was told that his real name sounded too Jewish/German, which could be fatal: if captured, he could be killed for being either a German traitor or Jewish. The army made him 'confident, self-reliant and with a sense of belief in [himself]'.[23] Because he entered a training programme to be an officer, he wasn't sent to the front during the war but was stationed in Germany in 1946 and later served in Northern Ireland.

On VE day, 13 May 1945, he was at the celebrations in central London but couldn't join in, feeling 'horrendously oppressed',[24] not knowing the fate of his family. The following year he accessed official files in Berlin, which noted that his parents and sister had been 'sent east'. He mistakenly took that to mean that they were killed in Auschwitz and he uncontrollably burst into tears visiting the concentration camp decades later in 1976. Eventually, he discovered their actual fate: in October 1942 they had been taken on a crowded three-day train journey from Berlin to Riga, the largest city in Latvia, led into the woods and shot.[25]

After the army, in 1947, Brent returned to Birmingham and, as an undergraduate student in zoology, began research with Medawar.

Already in the lab, Billingham, four years older than Brent, had been Medawar's first graduate student at Oxford after returning from active service in the navy. Impressed by the military rigour that Billingham brought to his planning and performing of experiments, Medawar obtained a position for him so that the two could move together from Oxford to Birmingham in 1947. Billingham came from a non-academic background – his father owned a fish and chip shop – and in general he was more down-to-earth, less of a philosopher, than Medawar. But Billingham's role in the team is not to be underestimated; he was ingenious at getting experiments to work technically and, Brent recalls, he had a 'single-minded dedication to his career'.[26]

In Birmingham, initially ignorant of Owen's earlier research, Medawar and Billingham performed experiments to test whether or not skin grafts could have a practical use in determining whether cattle twins were identical or non-identical. They did this as a small side project to give some immediate relevance to their work, since such a test would have particular significance for farmers in identifying female calves (called freemartins) that had become masculinized and sterile by being exposed to hormones from a non-identical male twin. Medawar and Billingham's test involved simply grafting skin from one animal to another and observing the outcome. They predicted that non-identical twins would reject grafts from each other, while identical twins would readily accept grafts. However, they were stunned to find out that cattle twins always accepted grafts from each other, no matter whether they were identical or not. The penny dropped when they eventually read Owen's earlier research, which had demonstrated that even non-identical cattle twins shared blood cells, presumably through a shared placenta. Transplants *could* work between genetically different animals, and from their experiments and Owen's earlier study, the trick seemed to be that, when animals shared tissue as a foetus, they could later in life still accept transplants from each other.

So the team of Billingham, Brent and Medawar – together in their new lab in London, 1951 – discussed a specific experimental plan that could test this idea. They decided that they could use inbred mice, which have defined genetic traits obtained by mating siblings many times. They injected cells from one inbred mouse strain directly into unborn foetal mice of another, non-identical, strain. They discovered that after birth, when tested as adults, the injected mice were able to accept skin from the unrelated mouse strain whose cells had been injected. These were startling, ground-breaking results – a solution to the ancient problem of transplantation. Jean dubbed the treated mice 'super-mice'.

The super-mice had become tolerant to skin grafts from unrelated mice whose cells they had been exposed to when foetuses. This was not the bolt from the blue that radioactivity was, for example – the trio had planned and carried out a specific experiment to test a hypothesis – but, as with radioactivity, it cannot be over-emphasized how important their discovery was; as with radioactivity, nothing in our everyday experience hints at the fact they discovered.

Key to their success as a team, all three were trained in zoology, so they spoke the same scientific language and, perhaps most important of all, they were all dedicated workaholics. Although this might read as though the breakthrough happened smoothly and simply, in practice the team had to go back and forth with variations in the conditions of the experiment to get things to work out. And in the midst of it all there was, of course, no guarantee it was ever going to work out. Doing science is like playing snakes and ladders: you can be five squares from glory, but the die rolls to four, lands you on a snake and you're back at square one. To win, the team worked long and hard.

They then went on to verify that the process was also true for other species – doing similar, but less extensive, experiments with chicken chicks. The transplantation problem had been solved, but in laboratory conditions, and using animals rather than humans. The team were acutely aware that this was not yet a practical medical advance: it would be impractical to inject cells into a human foetus. But their experiments had nevertheless revealed a solution to a problem previously thought insoluble. They had shown that it is, after all, possible to breach the natural barrier for transplantation between unrelated animals. In 2010 I met with Brent at his home in north London and asked what the trio's reactions were to this astonishing discovery. I had anticipated an answer involving some tension-releasing euphoria, but he simply replied, 'Well, we just worked harder.' Medawar and his team, I assume, would have subscribed to the view that Noël Coward put in a nutshell: 'Work is much more fun than fun.'

During these periods of intense research, Medawar didn't even buy his wife Jean birthday or Christmas presents – that would have taken up time. He simply asked her to go and buy whatever she wanted. And they even joked about her writing the tag: 'To my darling wife from her devoted husband'.[27] Medawar later recalled, perhaps not entirely joking, that he was 'an outstandingly rotten father and neglected [his four] children disgracefully ... due to [his] total preoccupation with research.'[28] Even within his team, Medawar was well aware of Brent's background but, despite sharing a great deal of time together, they never discussed the Holocaust or religion, or any other sensitive issue.[29]

After the mice experiments, the trio of Billingham, Brent and Medawar became stars in the scientific world, known in the US as 'the holy trinity'. In 1956 the trio published their *magnum opus*,[30] expanding the initial three and a half pages published in 1953 into fifty-seven pages of incredibly detailed analysis accompanied by twenty photos of experiments involving mice, chickens and a duck.[31] Then, in 1960, Medawar won the Nobel Prize, together with Burnet, the Australian scientist who, in parallel to Medawar's experiments, developed a theory that the immune system could learn not to react to cells and tissues present at the foetus stage of life. Medawar openly wished that the prize – awarded collectively to a maximum of three people – could have been awarded to all of his team.[32] And in a strong public statement of how important Billingham and Brent were, Medawar shared the prize money with them. In a personal letter to Brent's wife, Joanne, Medawar wrote that 'I wish to make it absolutely clear that it [a share of the prize money] is no way a present but comes to Leslie as of *right*.'[33]

Medawar was also generous to Ray Owen, who had made the early ground-breaking observation that blood cells can be transferred between non-identical cattle twins. Medawar wrote to Owen: 'Of the five or six hundred letters I have had about the Nobel Prize, yours is the one I most wanted to receive. I think it is very wrong that you are not sharing in this prize ... you started it all.'[34]

It is not simply winning a Nobel Prize that makes Medawar's name endure, it is also the brilliance of his essays and books, which remain influential; the eminent biologist and writer Richard Dawkins takes inspiration from Medawar as the 'wittiest scientist ever'.[35] An example of Medawar's incisive writing and clear thinking comes across well in his critique of a book, *The Phenomenon of Man* by French philosopher Pierre Teilhard de Chardin, published in 1955. The book, hugely influential at the time, used flowery language to present wild speculations about the process of evolution. 'It is the style [of the book],' Medawar wrote, 'that creates the illusion of content ... The greater part of it ... is nonsense, tricked out with a variety of tedious metaphysical conceits, and its author can be excused of dishonesty only on the grounds that before deceiving others he has taken great pains to deceive himself.'[36]

A year after Medawar's Nobel Prize came the death of another pioneering London-based transplantation scientist, Peter Gorer. Medawar wrote a memoir of him for the Royal Society. While Medawar's research linked transplantation to the body's immune response, Gorer's research had earlier connected transplantation to our compatibility genes, and some felt that he should have won the Nobel Prize.[37] But Gorer had not been a great communicator – he usually spoke with a cigarette hanging from his mouth – and probably the reception of his work suffered for it. He dressed carelessly, behaved eccentrically and regularly drank half a bottle of whisky in an evening.[38] He was undervalued even in his own institute, the rigid medical environment of Guy's Hospital in London, only being promoted to professor shortly before his death. While Medawar had given up smoking in light of Richard Doll's landmark 1950 paper linking smoking to lung cancer, Gorer died of the disease, aged fifty-four, when he could have been enjoying widespread recognition of his achievements. Gorer's research also probably came too early to be appreciated by the general public; his main discoveries were in the mid-1930s, and it was only later, during the Second World War, that surgery for the injured made plain the importance of research in transplantation.

Gorer had studied the length of time tumours survived in different breeds of mice. He injected tumour cells into mice and then observed whether the tumour would grow and kill the mouse or whether the tumour would be destroyed and the mouse survive. Publishing his key findings in 1936, aged just twenty-nine, he discovered that what happened to the tumour depended on whether the mouse in question had inherited a particular genetic component. If a recipient mouse had a different version of the genetic component, compared to the mouse from which the tumour was taken, the recipient mouse would be able to kill the transplanted tumour and survive. But if it had the same set of these genes as the mouse from which the tumour was originally taken, the transplanted tumour would grow and kill the mouse.

Then Gorer made an intellectual leap. This process, he suggested, was not particular to tumours. Although tumours are abnormal in their growth characteristics, they were behaving in these transplantation experiments just as any other tissue would. That is, the same rules for transplantation were obeyed both by tumours and by other tissues – so, Gorer postulated, his experiments had revealed the general rules for transplantation. In effect, he discovered a specific genetic component that determined whether or not cells transplanted from one mouse to another would be attacked or left alone. In time, it was found out that the genetic component identified by Gorer includes the mouse genes equivalent to our human compatibility genes; so Gorer's transplantation experiments are arguably where our knowledge of compatibility genes really began.

The relationship between Medawar and Gorer was complex. Medawar would often make jokes at Gorer's expense and they argued vigorously about several scientific issues. One long-running argument was over the nature of red blood cells in mice and humans – comparing experiments in these different species caused confusion because, as we now know, the protein encoded by compatibility genes is found in small amounts on mouse red blood cells but not at all on human ones – but they didn't know this at the time. Nevertheless, they retained an appreciation of each other's brilliance. Fellows of the Royal Society can submit a document to record the influences and inspiration for their achievements and Medawar was moved when he found out that Gorer had written of his 'close friendship with P. B. Medawar'. Gorer wrote that 'it is not easy to say how each [of us] influenced the other's ideas, but the influence was none the less potent'.[39]

In 1962, a year after Gorer's death, Medawar was appointed director at the National Institute of Medical Research in Mill Hill, London. Each day an institute chauffeur would collect him from his Hampstead home and take him to work; he was always there by 9 a.m., even following overnight flights back from the US. As this most celebrated period in Medawar's research career – with Billingham and Brent – drew to a close, he and Jean visited Russia at the invitation of the Soviet Academy of Sciences. In 1950s England, Jean's role as housewife was seen as perfectly normal; in Russia, however, she was commonly asked what her profession was. The question lingered in her mind, and when she returned to north London, Jean began to work in Islington's family planning clinic. She went on to become the second chair of the Family Planning Association in 1967, at a time when the contraceptive pill was radically changing attitudes to sex. But soon after, Jean and Peter's personal life changed dramatically and tragically.

On 7 September 1969, at the end of a week-long meeting of the British Science Association, a few weeks after Armstrong and Aldrin walked on the moon, Peter Medawar, as that year's president, gave a reading at Exeter Cathedral – as part of a tradition at the time for the Science Association to participate in an annual religious service. As he read from the Book of Solomon – 'For Wisdom is more mobile than any motion; because of her pureness she pervades and penetrates all things . . .' – his voice slurred suddenly. He slumped into his seat and fell unconscious. Jean later recalled that in a flash 'he had fallen from a pinnacle of achievements into a state very near death'. She knew instantly that he'd had a stroke.

For at least a year after his severe right-sided cerebral haemorrhage, Medawar was incapacitated. The head office of the Medical Research Council thought they should now replace him with a younger, fully fit leader for their prestigious institute. Many in the institute, including those close to Peter, agreed that this would be sensible. A young scientist, Liz Simpson, who had recently joined Medawar's team as a vet, had already taken over some of the day-to-day running of Medawar's projects, which continued to be important. They were testing, for example, whether or not giving drugs to suppress the immune system and aid transplantation success would have the side effect of allowing cancer to develop. Even Simpson thought it would be better for

Medawar to step down from his headship. But Peter and Jean were both stubborn about the issue. Jean especially fought the Medical Research Council, and Peter was kept on as head of the institute for another two years, even though he was paralysed down his left side, with his useless arm in a sling and his left leg in a splint. Eventually, under pressure from the Medical Research Council, he did step down, and moved in 1972 to head a transplantation biology department in a new clinical research centre at Northwick Park Hospital.

Even after two more debilitating strokes in the mid-1980s, it was clear that Medawar's compulsion to work remained undimmed. In a 1984 interview for *New Scientist* magazine, he remarked: 'I do nothing but work – ever . . . I'm not going to retire.'[40] Doctors looking at Peter's brain scan were astonished – they couldn't understand how he was able to have any life at all, let alone write books and work at Northwick Park Hospital each weekday. One positive outcome of his illness was that he was more often available for discussion in his laboratory[41] and became more accessible to his children at home.[42] One of his four children, Charles Medawar, said to me in 2010 that he has far more memories of his father after his stroke than before it.[43]

The eminent evolutionary scientist and writer Stephen Jay Gould remarked that Medawar 'lived far longer and better with half a body than the vast majority of people could ever hope to survive with all systems functional'.[44] And indeed, following his first stroke, Peter and Jean had eighteen productive years together, including the publication of two books as co-authors. Liz Simpson, who helped run things at the clinical research centre while Peter was ill, recalled that 'even 10 per cent of his mind was better than 100 per cent of most other people's'.[45]

Medawar died on 2 October 1987. His obituary in *Nature*, written by his protégé Avrion Mitchison, called him 'the most distinguished British biologist of his generation'.[46] To this day, Mitchison, a major scientific figure in his own right, lights up at the mention of Medawar, referring to him as 'magical'.[47] The primary importance of Medawar's scientific work is a given, but it is these testimonies and many others alike, as well the stream of books he published, that sealed the legend of Medawar. Oxford University and University College London have buildings named after Medawar. C. P. Snow, the novelist and physicist, proclaimed that 'If he [Medawar] had designed the world, it would be a better place.'[48]

Medawar – with his co-workers Billingham and Brent – had made the glorious discovery that transplantation tolerance could be achieved for any cells present in the foetus stage of development – so-called 'acquired tolerance'. Drawing on Gorer's research, they also knew that a genetic component was important in controlling transplantation compatibility. But they did not have a clear idea about what our compatibility genes really did. All that was apparent was that they were important for transplantation and that somehow transplant rejection was linked to the immune system. Towards the end of Medawar's life, a deeper understanding of compatibility genes in our immune system was emerging, but he died one week before another trio of scientists, this time at Harvard University, published an atomic-scale picture that vividly revealed how our compatibility genes work. Medawar would have loved it.

The day before his first stroke, Medawar ended his lecture with a quotation from the seventeenth-century philosopher Thomas Hobbes. Hobbes's writing struck a chord with Medawar in proclaiming that life is like a race and the most important thing is to be in it, to be fully engaged, ambitious and go-getting, to improve the world. Eighteen years later, that same quotation, 'There can be no contentment but in proceeding', was engraved on his headstone.[49] Jean died in 2005 and is buried next to him.

Medawar could not have known the full impact of his work, reaching far beyond transplantation and immunology. Yet it has also become clear that many problems in medicine are not scientific; they are social, ethical and even economical. His son Charles established an organization, the Social Audit, which evolved into a significant force aiming to hold pharmaceutical companies to account. In its heyday in the 1990s, Charles's web pages had a million visitors per year[50] and brought attention to problems such as how some drugs were being marketed unnecessarily in the Global South.

Billingham died in 2002; the last years of his life being made miserable by Parkinson's disease.[51] Brent is the last surviving member of the 'holy trinity' – the only domino still standing, as he puts it.[52] In his mid-eighties, he still actively pursues transplantation research, working within a large European consortium of labs looking at new ways to suppress immune responses in kidney transplantation, something that remains a considerable issue today: about 85 per cent of people in the UK needing an organ transplant are waiting for a kidney.[53] Brent had started his long career by performing experiments that led to a Nobel Prize for his PhD supervisor, a prize Medawar shared with the Australian Macfarlane Burnet, who developed theories independently that ended up being vindicated by the holy trinity's experiments. It's Burnet whom we need to turn to next. From the other side of the world, his ideas deepened our understanding of the holy trinity's experiments and gave a new answer to why we are ever so slightly and ever so importantly different from each other.

Frank Macfarlane Burnet

2

Self / Non-self

It is well established that electrons and protons whirl in every atom; packs of atoms assemble in every molecule; societies of molecules create cells; and your body is a metropolis of cells. So, are we all essentially the same? No. Medawar's story of graft rejection showed that my body can tell apart my cells from yours. Recall that his patients' bodies could only accept skin grafted from elsewhere on their own bodies; skin taken from the bodies of others, even relatives, was rejected. How can this be? What molecular substance gives each of us our individuality and how could our bodies distinguish it? And this is where Frank Macfarlane Burnet moves things forward – by asking: how does our body know its tissues and cells as its own? Or, put another way, how does the human body discriminate *self* from *non-self*?

Burnet was an introvert; 'a fairly humourless dry old stick who wouldn't let his hair down – the opposite of Medawar', Leslie Brent recalls.[1] But he is also one of the greatest thinkers there has ever been in human biology. In 1937, aged thirty-eight, Burnet formulated the idea that discriminating between what's you and what's not you is the immune system's *raison d'être,* that recognizing and destroying substances that are non-self is precisely what the immune system must do. And from this Burnet realized that the problem of how our body recognizes disease is part and parcel of understanding how our body knows its own cells and tissues.

This huge step forward in understanding how our immune system works descends directly from the simple fact that disease can be caused by germs. Beyond its obvious practical importance, knowledge of germs helped us to understand that disease is caused by something outside of us, something *non-self*. Although we all now know that germs cause disease, this fact took millennia to establish. Indeed, the history of how humans have struggled to understand disease is important in illustrating how revolutionary Burnet's ideas really were.

The Greek philosopher and physician Hippocrates, born around 460 BCE, is considered the first to have suggested that disease is not a direct act of God, or an outcome from some superstitious belief, but that instead it has a natural cause. Greek physicians, and later the Romans, took as fact that disease came about from an excess or deficiency of one of four 'humours' – black bile, yellow bile, phlegm and blood – each of which had to be present at the right levels for us to be healthy. This view endured, essentially unchanged, for two millennia.[2]

A description of disease is not mere semantics: past misunderstandings have brought out the worst in human behaviour. When the Black Death arrived in Europe in 1347, a true understanding of disease was still centuries away, and the beliefs of the age had grave consequences. Estimates put deaths caused by the plague at anywhere between 75 and 200 million, slashing Europe's population by at least a third, and possibly half. It would return in waves – though never again to such catastrophic effect – for the next 400 years. Inevitably, crowded cities were worst hit: half the populations of Paris and London perished. Chroniclers of the time said the living were scarcely able to bury the dead; that the devastation seemed more final than Noah's flood.[3] Doctors had only opinions, not facts, to explain what was going on. Most people believed that humanity was being punished by God, while astrologers asserted that the horror was caused by an alignment of planets Mars, Saturn and Jupiter (even though this doesn't seem able to explain why only some people succumbed to the plague).

A belief that the plague was caused by sins against God twisted into a desire to kill the enemies of Christ. One common belief was that the Black Death was spread by Jews and other non-Christians. Jews were accused of poisoning water wells in an attack against Christianity, and often confessed to this under torture. In vengeance, thousands were murdered in cities across France, Austria and Germany. The sentiment helped seed the following century's Spanish Inquisition. A lack of understanding about the nature of disease played a role in allowing

European leaders to force religious conversion and burn people at the stake. The painful irony is it that a contemporary understanding of disease reveals that human genetic variation is central to our immune defences.

A modern view of disease begins in the nineteenth century, the giants of the era being Charles Darwin and the French microbiologist Louis Pasteur. The two legends never met face-to-face, alas, though it would have been possible. Today, Pasteur gets his name onto almost every packet of cheese, while Darwin is revered, sometimes cursed, for his supposed slaying of God. Pasteur first showed that living cells were essential for making wine and then that a similar budding and multiplying of cells occurred in soured milk. At the time, it was hotly disputed whether fermentation was some kind of mechanical break- down of chemicals or a biological process. Pasteur clarified that minuscule living organisms, unseen by the human eye, were at the heart of these phenomena. But his brilliance was in realizing that we, too, must be exposed to this new-found world of invisible organisms. Since unseen microbes can cause dramatic changes to the nature of things – as in fermentation – he postulated that these unseen microbes might also underlie human disease. Many thought this a ridiculous idea: how could something so small that it can't be seen kill some- thing so much more powerful like us?

Pasteur's ideas about microscopic organisms highlighted a major problem: at the time, nobody knew where minuscule living organisms came from. Could minute life-forms arise from spontaneous chemical reactions when milk goes sour, or when maggots appear in rotting meat, or does life really only ever arise from pre-existing life? For the prestigious French Académie des Sciences, this was the most pressing issue of the day. Pasteur settled the debate with an ingenious simple experiment.

He took a glass flask and shaped its neck into a thin tube bent to an s-shaped curve. To this so-called swan-neck flask he added a clear broth, similar to a soup base, which had been heated to kill off all liv- ing things. Although the broth was exposed to the air through the s-shaped neck, nothing would grow in the liquid – microbes and dust particles from the air would collect in the curve of the flask's neck and not reach the broth. But after Pasteur then broke off the curved neck, the broth would turn cloudy – things now started to grow. Microbes had fallen into the broth from dust in the air. So, life does not spontaneously arise in the broth, it falls in from the air. But another, more subtle implication was that minute organisms are all around us.

That such minute organisms can cause disease in humans was finally established in 1876 by the German scientist and medical doctor Robert Koch, son of a mining engineer. Koch set up a makeshift laboratory in his four-room flat while working as the district medical officer in Wollstein, Western Poland, isolated from libraries and other scientists and without financial support for research, simply using equipment he purchased himself – apart from his microscope, which was a present from his wife. By day he saw his medical patients; out of hours he worked on mice, infecting them with anthrax bacteria that he obtained from the spleens of dead farm animals.

It was already known that organs or blood from an infected animal could pass on the disease. But one of Koch's brilliant experiments was to culture some of the rod-shaped anthrax bacteria in the fluid from an ox's eye, and to demonstrate that these cultured, isolated bacteria could still give mice the disease. In this way Koch established, once and for all, that bacteria can cause disease. In fact, we now know there are about 5×10^{32} bacteria on earth. It no longer seems ridiculous that minuscule unseen germs could harm us. Now the more astonishing thing is that our immune system is, more often than not, actually able to protect us.

Koch's and Pasteur's discoveries complement each other perfectly but personally they were arch-enemies. For much of their careers, they fired off at each other vicious patriotic claims for their own discoveries, mirroring the Franco-German political disputes of the time.[4] Koch, younger by twenty years, suggested that Pasteur could not obtain microbes as pure as he could, and that Pasteur's experiments were usually meaningless. At a meeting in Geneva in 1882, Pasteur, by then aged sixty, directed a barbed observation at Koch, who was seated in the front row. Describing his latest experiments with chicken cholera, which showed that the disease-causing bacteria could be attenuated and used as a vaccine, Pasteur then noted, 'However blazingly clear the demonstrated truth, it has not always had the privilege of being easily accepted.' Just to make absolutely clear who he was talking about, he continued: 'Dr Koch, who finds nothing remarkable in this experiment . . . does not believe that I operated as I said I did, with eighty chickens . . . because that would have cost too much money.' Sitting with his students, Koch listened unmoved to Pasteur's nationalist punchline: 'But in view of establishing this great fact . . . my government allowed me not to worry about the expense.'[5]

The following year, an editorial in the *Boston Medical and Surgical Journal* wrote about the debacle with a timeless wisdom that can be transposed to any number of disputes:

> It is to be regretted that abstract questions of scientific truth or error cannot be divorced from the personalities of discoverers and wrangling over priority, and that such anger should possess celestial minds. The expanse of the unknown is broad enough for all voyagers to pursue their way without collision.[6]

But perhaps these words are naive. Pioneers in science, or anything else, must be strong-willed enough to travel in a new direction and thick-skinned enough to withstand criticism from guardians of the prevailing dogma. A level of inner confidence that gets very close to arrogance is often of benefit to any trailblazer; self-belief is as critical as talent.

To relate to this kind of almost stereotyped conflict between scientists it's important to remember that, while artists are able to delight in their individual output being individual, scientists never really produce anything unique. They can only be first in uncovering information that otherwise would have been discovered by somebody else later. In the end both Pasteur and Koch, as well as many others, contributed to the discovery that germs cause disease. Koch won the Nobel Prize in 1905, but Pasteur had died six years before the first Nobel Prizes were awarded. Both have major institutes named after them today.

The concept of germs is so deeply implanted in us today that it takes effort to appreciate that the idea that so small a thing could be so harmful was initially thought ridiculous. It had to be explicitly proven that disease was not caused by the wrath of evil spirits, or an imbalance of black bile, yellow bile, phlegm and blood, or a poisonous vapour from decaying matter (as in the so-called miasma theory of the Middle Ages). Distinct diseases do have different origins, but many are caused by minuscule microbes, and realizing this is undoubtedly one of the greatest triumphs of the second millennium.

Sanitation and hygiene, as well as almost all of modern medicine, builds on this basic premise. Indeed, in *Life* magazine's list of the top 100 most important events in the last millennium, the discovery of germs ranked sixth. Gutenberg's printing of the Bible came out top, but the existence of germs beats vaccination (thirteenth), evolution (fifteenth), the telephone (twentieth), penicillin (twenty-second), landing on the moon (thirty-third) and the structure of DNA (seventy-sixth).[7] Such a list is highly subjective – the 'discovery' of Coca-Cola was a surprising choice, to say the least, as the eighty-second most important event in a thousand years – but unquestionably, the sixth choice was good: nothing has done more for our well-being than the epochal discovery of germs. This was also an essential first step towards the important idea that our immune system can defend us by discriminating between our own cells and tissues, i.e. 'self', and every other thing out there, i.e. 'non-self'.

Of course, the language of self and non-self has connotations far beyond our immune system. Many philosophers and religious scholars have discussed the meaning of self as a metaphysical concept as well as in terms of our physical body. Buddha, for instance, discusses self and non-self a lot. Buddha refers to non-self, or not-self, as things perceived by our senses that we must not cling to, while self is the part of us which seeks pleasure, lusts after vanity, brings about envy and gives rise to hatred. The very existence of self, Buddha teaches, is nothing more than an illusion, and we must strive in our lives to be free of this mirage. Such holistic and spiritual interpretations of 'self' are simply from different realms of thinking to the molecular description of 'self' that immunology provides. Using the language of 'self' and 'non-self' in describing ideas about the molecules that comprise our bodies is provocative and yet, at some level, individuality surely *is* constructed from our constituent chemistry.

Burnet started using the terminology of 'self' and 'non-self' in 1940. Comparatively isolated from any international hub of scientific activity like Medawar's base in war-torn London, he first used the terms in a loose metaphorical sense, but by 1949 he and his Australian colleague Frank Fenner, fifteen years younger than Burnet, set out their view clearly – in what they called the self-marker hypothesis – that the human immune system works by discriminating its own self from non-self.[8]

Fenner humbly maintained that in this work he was merely a junior assistant checking a few facts, that 'Burnet was responsible for all the interpretation and speculation'.[9] In fact, Fenner went on to publish over 300 scientific papers and he played a considerable role in the eradication of smallpox.[10] And throughout his stellar career, he always kept a photo of Burnet on his desk.[11]

Quite different from Medawar, Burnet was not driven to solve the clinically important problem of transplantation. Burnet never experienced the shock of pacing a war wounds hospital as Medawar did, and Burnet never collected clinical data himself. Though he had previously studied viruses and had made important experimental discoveries regarding how influenza spread, what drove him was the desire to understand what happened during an immune response: in fact, his burning ambition was to discover a grand unified theory of immunology.

In this respect, Burnet was following in giant footsteps. He was twenty-two when Albert Einstein won the Nobel Prize, and Richard Feynman, a dominant force in physics, was a contemporary of him and Medawar. Both Einstein and Feynman were obsessed with the quest for fundamental laws that unify the different forces in nature. That way of thinking continues today – Stephen Hawking and many others freely talk of our search for a grand unified theory of everything – and Burnet was of the same ilk.

As with his hero Charles Darwin a century earlier, collecting beetles – a vivid portrait of biological diversity – sowed the seeds of Burnet's tenacious search for generalizations and underlying principles. He made copious notes on unusual beetle behaviours and filled sketch books with drawings of beetle legs and antennae.[12] Later in life, after dinners with his family, he would often read the current issues of the scientific journals *Nature* and *Science* and keep copious records of what he read on small cards.[13]

It is likely that he found this solace in collecting and organizing, at least in part, because he never established a deep relationship with his parents.[14] His mother was preoccupied with caring for his mentally disabled elder sister Doris and as a result became very reclusive. His father spent little time with the family, preferring to be out with friends, playing golf or trout fishing, and Burnet later recalled that, even as young as eight, he disapproved of some of his father's deals as the local bank manager.[15] Burnet's sister's disability, resulting from complications at birth, was not allowed to be discussed outside the family, and friends were discouraged from coming over to play. Perhaps this contributed to him growing up to be shy and introspective – 'always something of a solitary', he said of himself.[16] By age seven, Burnet had already won a prize for academic achievement at school and he later graduated as the second-top student in Medicine at the University of Melbourne.[17] He loved the wealth of the Melbourne Public Library – especially all the 'knowledge enshrined there about the anatomy of beetles'.[18]

On the evening of 21 October 1921, he heard his father was seriously ill back at the family home in Terang, a small town of around 2,000 residents just over 200 kilometres south-west of Melbourne. The next day, Burnet rushed back to Terang by train with the intention of laying to rest the strain in their distant relationship, but it was too late.

One thing Burnet learned from his father was patriotism; in part a reaction against Australia being seen as an English colony. It was always important for Burnet to prove that Australian science could stand up to be as good as science anywhere else in the world.[19] In 1944, based on his early success studying viruses, he was offered a lucrative position at Harvard University, which offered a research environment that far surpassed Melbourne, but he turned it down because he thought that his children should grow up in Australia.[20]

Burnet had been especially shy with women, and danced with a girl for the first time aged twenty-four. Soon after, he met his future wife Linda through an arranged introduction. Like Jean Medawar, Linda accepted his need to work hard and to be left alone often. Despite eventually being thrust into the limelight as a Nobel laureate and director of a prestigious institute, he always kept his family life very private. In his autobiography, published in 1968, he wrote of Linda that 'beyond recording that we were married on 10 July 1928, I shall say nothing more directly about her'.[21] The eldest of their three children, Elizabeth

Dexter, recalled in 2011 that Linda would commonly 'fob off anyone that threatened to disrupt his work':[22] 'He could never say no, but she could!'[23] Just like Medawar, Burnet was shielded from distractions by his wife, who saw her role defined by having a husband capable of immensely important discoveries.

Burnet, like Medawar again, was especially influenced by Ray Owen's experiments. Owen, we recall, discovered that cattle twins in a non-identical pair are tolerant to cells from each other, presumably because of a shared placenta.[24] In fact, the seminal importance of Owen's work was little recognized until Burnet and Fenner highlighted it in their 1949 publication – Medawar, for example, wasn't even aware of Owen's work until he read about it in Burnet and Fenner's paper.[25]

Building on Owen's discovery, Burnet speculated that the twins' tolerance for each other must have developed by the calves being exposed to the other's cells when foetuses. From this, he went on to suggest that the human immune system must also learn to recognize our own cells and tissues when foetuses or in early childhood. They didn't understand how this could work in any detail but it just seemed to make sense that the immune system would learn what our body is made of at an early age so that it is then ready to attack anything else.

Burnet had no proof of this hypothesis, and in 1949 could only conclude that 'it remains to be seen whether this concept is of value'.[26] It was a few years later that Medawar's skin grafting experiments, essentially those three and a half pages reported in 1953, showed these ideas to be right: that the immune system would indeed become tolerant to any cells or tissues present early on in an animal's life.

Although this won Burnet and Medawar the Nobel Prize in 1960, nobody had any idea how this really worked: how did the immune system learn to recognize the body's own cells and tissues early in life? Indeed, Burnet considered this Nobel-Prize-winning achievement as being 'essentially only a way-station on the road to the broader conception' of how the immune system worked.[27] He was right: his next theory has claim to being far more important than that which won him the Nobel Prize.

The focus of Burnet's thinking, and that of many of his contemporaries, was antibodies. Discovered in 1890, antibodies are soluble

31

proteins found in blood that stick to and neutralize all kinds of germs and potentially dangerous molecules. The key problem lay in understanding how such antibodies could recognize so many different kinds of germs, while seemingly not triggering an attack on our own cells or tissue. And here's the really big mystery: by the mid-1950s, while chemists over the world were starting to synthesize new molecules that had never existed before, biologists found that the human body is able to make antibodies that recognize and stick to these brand-new molecules. It's one thing to try and work out how antibodies could recognize specific germs, but here was evidence that in fact antibodies can recognize anything, even brand-new molecules that have never existed in the universe before. How could this work? Everyone agreed that this was the greatest problem in our understanding of how our immune system worked: how could antibodies react to a potentially limitless number of 'non-self' molecules but still not mount an attack on 'self' cells and tissues?

The prevalent view, led by the two-time Nobel-Prize-winning American biochemist Linus Pauling, was that antibodies could mould into any shape to fit around foreign molecules and trigger their destruction. This was the so-called 'instructional theory': a generic antibody is instructed by the foreign molecule to fit around it. London-born Danish scientist Niels Jerne, who went on to win the Nobel Prize for Medicine in 1984, didn't like this idea at all.

Jerne was a late developer in science. He grew up in the Netherlands and studied physics at the University of Leiden, but he then spent thirteen years in various occupations before deciding to return to academic study, this time medicine, and eventually he obtained a PhD in Copenhagen in 1951, aged nearly forty. After his PhD, while working in Copenhagen at the Danish National Serum Institute, a government research institute for infectious diseases, Jerne thought about the antibody problem. For much of his life before that time he had considered himself in a 'dark middle age'[28] – certainly not thinking about immunology. Even so, it is telling that, throughout his life, he saved nearly all his correspondence and manuscripts in anticipation that one day they would be important – confident that his life would be of widespread interest in the end.

Prior to thinking about antibodies, Jerne had many difficulties in his life.[29] Sexually, he was keen on sadomasochism, but it is not clear if he shared this tendency with his wife Tjek. They bonded through their passion to live free from the shackles of social convention; but both had extra-marital affairs and their relationship suffered as a result. Tjek was a very successful artist in Copenhagen and she struggled with everyday difficulties raising their two children while Jerne was often absent, working in his father's Danish bacon business. In 1945, Tjek committed suicide. Jerne struggled with guilt: he had threatened Tjek with divorce. Immersion in science – and specifically antibodies – may have been his escape.[30]

Now that he had found something to focus his mind on, Jerne felt that the implication that any molecule at all could instruct cells how to make a well-suited antibody just seemed 'odd'.[31] There were also some more specific issues that worried Jerne, such as how an antibody could know which molecule it should fold around among all the components of a cell – why would antibodies only fold around non-self molecules?

Then one day, some nine years after his wife's suicide and four years after the publication of Burnet's paper, Jerne had a moment of inspiration on his way home from work. During his brisk twenty-minute walk, he formulated a new theory for how self and non-self discrimination worked.[32] He suddenly thought to himself that maybe all different shapes of antibody exist beforehand – a whole collection of differently shaped antibodies just circulating in the blood before any germ has been seen – so that any particular foreign molecule will be recognized by at least one of the pre-existing shapes of antibody. This would become known as 'selectionist theory', because there would be an antibody that could be selected from the pool of all the differently shaped antibodies, able to stick to the foreign molecule, leading to the molecule's destruction. Immediately, Jerne thought his theory had to be correct.[33]

James Watson, the scientist celebrated for his work with Francis Crick on the double helix shape of DNA, had come as a student in 1950 to work with Jerne at the Danish National Serum Institute, and the two had remained friends ever since. Watson listened carefully to Jerne's idea about antibodies and decided that it stank.[34] Pauling similarly dismissed it without hesitation.[35] Both thought the idea wrong because their practical experience of studying the shapes of molecules suggested to them that there simply couldn't be such an enormous pool of differently shaped antibodies pre-existing in our blood.

Burnet, however – lacking practical experience in examining the shapes of molecules – responded differently. He was immediately excited by the idea and – theoretically – realized it could be correct. He considered Jerne 'the most intelligent immunologist alive'[36] and, thinking deeply about his theory, came up with a crucial modification, which Jerne described as another 'guess'. Burnet presented his ideas concisely in two pages in his paper 'A modification of Jerne's theory of antibody production using the concept of clonal selection', published in the *Australian Journal of Science* in 1957, when he was aged fifty-seven – somewhat older than when scientists are usually thought to have their best, ground-breaking idea.[37]

Burnet's 'modification' to Jerne's theory was hugely important. It single-handedly transformed the reputation of both men – this was still three years before Burnet won the Nobel Prize with Medawar – and changed Jerne's original idea from one that 'stank' to one that has become a cornerstone in understanding how everything works in the immune system. In general, scientific papers do well to be remembered a few years after publication, but in this case, on the fiftieth anniversary of Burnet's paper, today's leading specialist journal *Nature Immunology* remarked on its exceptional significance: 'rarely has a field as large and influential been gathered together and encapsulated in so spare a form'.[38]

Burnet's modification was that the focus should be on the cells that make antibodies rather than the antibodies themselves.[39] Burnet speculated that one cell makes one particular shape of antibody and that all our antibody-making immune cells together make an unimaginably vast repertoire of 10 billion antibodies, each having a slightly different shape. So, for any particular non-self molecule that enters the body, at least one immune cell will make an antibody that is the right shape to stick to that particular molecule. When a cell sees a molecule that its antibodies can stick to, it multiplies, and lots of clones of the initial cell can then secrete the right antibody in bulk, efficiently neutralizing the dangerous molecule or germ. Burnet named the idea Clonal Selection Theory.[40]

Around the same time, American immunologist David Talmage, from the University of Colorado, published some related ideas. Yet, in a controversy that endures to this day, Burnet's legacy has put Talmage's contribution in the shade. It is a situation comparable to that of the Welsh-born naturalist Alfred Russel Wallace and his contemporary Charles Darwin, a century earlier. In June 1958, Wallace sent Darwin a twenty-odd-page letter detailing his ideas on how species can diverge as a result of environmental pressures. Darwin had independently been accumulating evidence for this idea over decades and the letter spurred him on to complete his book-length treatise on the idea, *On the Origin of Species*, published on 24 November 1859. Likewise, in 1956, Talmage sent Burnet an advance copy of his paper with his own ideas similar to Burnet's Clonal Selection Theory. Talmage had been inspired by Burnet and Fenner's 1949 paper describing the immune system as discriminating self and non-self.[41] Burnet, however, had already come to the same conclusions independently, and – again reminiscent of Darwin's primacy over Wallace – there is no doubt that he had explored the implications of the theory more completely.[42] In any case, almost everyone rejected the idea at first – Talmage puts it down to a general scepticism that all new ideas are judged by.[43]

The dominant argument against Burnet and Talmage was: why should immune cells make an enormous array of pre-existing antibodies able to recognize all manner of non-self molecules, most of which would never be used? It seemed wasteful and counter-productive. Yet for Burnet the idea was self-evident: simply put, it was Darwinian selection applied to cells inside our bodies. Indeed, Burnet viewed the human body like an ecosystem – a dynamic place where cells interact and can multiply or die. From this perspective, he envisaged that the cells in our immune system best suited to fight a particular germ could be activated to multiply and become a greater fraction of the total population of antibody-secreting cells.

In 1957, Gustav Nossal, a confident twenty-six-year-old Austrian medic working in the Hall Institute, Melbourne, suggested to the fifty-eight-year-old Burnet that he could easily disprove his 'pretty crazy theory' of clonal selection by showing that a single cell could actually make more than just one shape of antibody.[44] Nossal had just recently arrived in Melbourne, with his wife and new baby, to study for a PhD, having studied medicine in Sydney. To Nossal's surprise, Burnet was both excited and encouraging, and this was the beginning of a long collaboration between them. Over the years, Nossal learned that it worked best to never bluntly disagree with Burnet, and it paid great dividends to always subtly acknowledge his primacy.[45]

In 1957, Burnet didn't only encourage Nossal in his idea but also found him help with the experiment, in the form of US scientist Josh Lederberg. Lederberg, son of an orthodox Rabbi, was thirty-two, just six years older than Nossal, but he was already renowned for his pioneering research in the genetics of bacteria and was soon to win the Nobel Prize in 1958. Lederberg arrived at the Hall Institute in 1957 for a three-month sabbatical to work with Burnet, who suggested that he help Nossal. Excited by Nossal's idea, Lederberg taught him how to use a micromanipulator, a tool that allows you to move and manipulate objects under a microscope. The micromanipulator, it turned out, was the key to isolating individual antibody-secreting cells in separate liquid drops – a process crucial to the experiment Nossal was about to carry out.

Joshua

In the end, the actual breakthrough happened late in 1957, when Lederberg had already returned to the US. Nossal injected rats with two different strains of bacteria. He then isolated the antibody-secreting cells from the infected rats in droplets and watched when he added bacteria. His aim was to detect whether a single cell could stop the movement of one or both types of bacteria. What he found was that, while many of the single cells were able to stop one of the strains of bacteria moving, none of the single cell droplets had antibodies that could stop both.

This was a huge step. It showed that a single cell was capable of neutralizing only one type of bacteria – so a single cell must make just one shape of antibody.[46] This was the first experiment that really helped Burnet gain acceptance for his Clonal Selection Theory – the theory that an individual cell will be activated to multiply when that cell is the one that makes the right-shaped antibody to neutralize a problematic germ.

Subsequently, Nossal became as close to the self-contained, distant Burnet as anybody did in the institute: a friendship based on mutual intellectual respect. And Burnet nominated the precocious Nossal his successor as head of the Hall Institute, a post he assumed in 1965 at the age of thirty-five. Nossal was outgoing, entrepreneurial, a gifted speaker and a very successful leader. While the institute had an annual income of 350,000 Australian dollars when Burnet had left in 1965, Nossal had increased this to over 25 million by 1992.[47]

After he retired as director of the Hall Institute, Burnet became much more outspoken on broad issues such as ageing, the limits of medicine and the future of humanity.[48] He wrote books that didn't simply aim at making science accessible, but set out to answer big philosophical questions. To the surprise of many, given his constant and ongoing fear of speaking in public – which would often bring on migraines before interviews – he became Australia's leading scientific spokesperson.[49] In his penultimate book, published in 1978, Burnet's views were particularly uncompromising. While acknowledging the anathema of Hitler's racist policies, he wrote sympathetically about the underlying principles of eugenics. He spoke coolly and dispassionately about infanticide and euthanasia. His motive was a 'compassion to those individuals predestined to intolerable life' and not 'the idea of producing a better human species'.[50]

In 1969, a few years after Burnet retired from leading the Hall Institute, his wife Linda was diagnosed with lymphoid leukaemia, and from then on Burnet refused any offers to lecture abroad. After her death in November 1973, Burnet, devastated and isolated, found solace once again in collecting beetles, and he secretly wrote letters addressed to Linda every Sunday evening.[51] In 1976, he married a second time and subsequently expanded his public engagements.

Burnet died of cancer on 31 August 1985, comfortable that his discoveries would survive him. A staunch atheist, he had no time for any religious opinion about what happens when you die. Talmage wrote that Burnet was 'a dominant figure in immunology and medical science for half a century',[52] and Leslie Brent remarked that he was 'one of the deepest thinkers immunology has produced.'[53] Today, Burnet is remembered for Clonal Selection Theory far more than his Nobel-Prize-winning understanding of Medawar's experiments in acquired tolerance. But the details of how Burnet's theories really worked were left to others to sort out. For example, he didn't really know how each cell could make a differently shaped antibody.

At the time that Burnet formulated his theory, Crick, Watson and others had already worked out that a single gene encoded the instruction to make a single protein. Nossal's experiment showed that one cell made one specific shape of antibody, which backed up Burnet's idea, but raised the problem of how. That is, how could antibody-making cells each make differently shaped antibodies? The number of different shapes of antibodies in the human immune system – estimated to be 10–100 billion – far outstrips the number of genes we have – 25,000. So, how could each cell make a differently shaped antibody when it's impossible that each variation of antibody shape could be simply encoded in a gene?

This problem never stopped Burnet thinking that he had the right general principle; he just thought of it as a detail which remained to be understood. Eventually the problem was solved in a series of experiments beginning in the mid-1970s by Japanese-born Susumu Tonegawa, who won the Nobel Prize for this in 1987. The details deserve a whole other book, but in essence Tonegawa discovered (of course building on the work of many others) that antibody genes come in bits that join together in myriad ways. Normally, our genes never get altered in this way. But as each antibody-secreting cell develops in our bone marrow they rearrange these gene segments so that each cell ends up being able to make one antibody – one that's slightly different from those made by other cells.

But there was a second huge problem with Burnet's conception of the immune system. Burnet's Nobel-Prize-winning theory of acquired tolerance – as vindicated by Medawar's experiments – stated that the immune system learned to not react against our own cells and tissues. Again, what is extraordinary about Burnet's theory is that he was able to hit upon the right principle even though he could not have initially understood how the process took place in the body.

Insight into how acquired tolerance really works was achieved in 1961 by Jacques Miller, while he was studying for his PhD at the Chester Beatty Research Institute, London. Miller – along with several of his contemporaries – discovered the importance of the thymus, an organ above the heart previously thought to be entirely uninteresting. Containing many dead immune cells, the thymus had simply been written off as the place where cells went to die – a graveyard for immune cells. Miller, however, had a hunch that the thymus was rather more significant.

Far more important than what he set out to study – a particular leukaemia-causing virus – Miller observed that mice with their thymus removed very early in life were unable to fight off all kinds of infections. He immediately grasped the significance of this and then, in skin-graft experiments similar to those done by Medawar, Miller found that mice lacking their thymus could not reject genetically different skin. The thymus, Miller established, was not useless at all – it was crucial for establishing the mouse immune system, and, without it, mice couldn't fight infections or reject transplanted skin.

But not everyone was convinced. Even after reading Miller's publications, Medawar himself wrote that 'we shall come to regard the presence of lymphocytes [i.e. immune cells] in the thymus as an evolutionary accident of no very great significance'.[54] Medawar and many other scientific leaders of the time thought, quite simply: how on earth could an organ containing large numbers of dead cells be so vitally important in the creation of the immune system?

Burnet was an exception – he quickly grasped the importance of Miller's results. In a lecture he gave in London in June 1962, soon after Miller had published his research, Burnet suggested that there are so many dead cells in the thymus because they are all the immune cells that were killed off deliberately because they can be activated by 'self' molecules. In this way, Burnet suggested, the thymus is crucial to how the immune system discriminates between self and non-self: only immune cells that don't react to the body's own cells and tissues are let out of the thymus alive – and anything recognized by an immune cell that has made it out of the thymus must be something that has never been in your body before.

Pulling all these findings together, we begin to see how Burnet's theories really work in the body: first, immune cells shuffle segments of genes to define what each immune cell can react against. The outcome of this is that each individual immune cell reacts to a particular shape of molecule, say one found on a germ. However, this reactivity develops randomly, so initially all kinds of immune cells are produced, and some could react to your own cells or tissues. But before an immune cell is let out to patrol the body, the thymus checks that it won't react to the body's own cells and tissues. Any that can react to 'self' are killed off in the thymus and the rest are let out to defend. An immune cell, now out of the thymus and patrolling the body, seeing a particular germ, is activated to multiply and mounts our defence.

There are, in fact, two different types of immune cells in humans and many animals that rearrange their genes in this special way. Max Cooper at the University of Alabama was one scientist who helped establish this by showing that excision of different organs in birds led to losses in different types of immune cells.[55] These different types of immune cells became known as B cells and T cells. B cells are the antibody-secreting cells, named for their development in humans in bone marrow, while T cells are named for being the cells that pass through the thymus in their development.

Without doubt, the research by Burnet, Medawar and their contemporaries was a scientific revolution – one that had been over eighty years in the making, since Pasteur and Koch first established the existence of germs,[56] but which moved rapidly in its final stages during the 1950s and early '60s. From this revolution, major principles for how our body fights disease were established in an explosive synergy between experiments and ideas across three continents: Europe, the US and Australia. Today, acquired tolerance and clonal selection remain central to the understanding of the immune system. They are beautiful aspects of our inner anatomy; hidden from view but as elemental to our well-being as the circulation of blood.

Surprisingly, despite their partnership in establishing this scientific revolution, Burnet and Medawar met only rarely in person. International travel in those decades was relatively uncommon, and Burnet was fifty before he travelled overseas to a scientific conference.[57] Their interactions came largely through their formal scientific publications. Even here, their exchange of ideas did not develop systematically. It is tempting – but incorrect – to imagine that Burnet published a hypothesis that Medawar followed up with experiments: the idealized, so-called hypothetico-deductive model of how science works. Medawar himself was very critical of this view of science.[58] How any idea develops between people is complicated, and paradigm-changing science is no exception. New knowledge is never attained in a coherent linear sequence of events: only a twisted path leads to something you couldn't see from the start.

This revolution came from a number of people thinking about the immune system in different ways – each with their own motives and perspective – and the fundamentals of immunology were established only when their contributions were put together. And these basic rules of our immune system were revealed long before much was known about the underlying molecular details. As we've seen, Burnet and Jerne developed a number of general principles that proved to be right even though there was very little knowledge available about the actual cells and molecules involved in the human immune system. Similarly, Medawar's experiments were at the level of physiology rather than in the minutiae of how the immune system worked. This is the opposite way round to how most biological research works now.

Today, we have the tools to be able to manipulate genes and proteins in cells and animals. It's more common, therefore, to first identify the genetic or molecular requirements of a cell's behaviour, with general principles being built up afterwards. For example, the way in which cells divide, the subject of a Nobel Prize won by Leland Hartwell, Tim Hunt and Paul Nurse in 2001, was worked out through identification of the molecules and proteins that control the process. This in turn led to the idea that cells move through stages and checkpoints as they divide in two – the cell cycle – and deregulation of this sequence of events can lead to tumour formation. But the likes of Burnet and Medawar worked in a different era of biological science, before genes and proteins could be easily manipulated, which surely adds to the magnitude of their achievements. Theirs was a glorious age when big concepts opened up about the immune system, and the details were left for others to fathom.

3

Dead but Alive in Parts

Burnet and Medawar, and others, together established that the recognition of self and non-self can be reduced, in essence, to the fact that immune cells reactive to self are eliminated early in life. But what practical importance does this insight have? The immediate impact of Medawar's and Burnet's insights – especially Medawar's – was in changing people's perceptions of why transplantation often failed. They revealed, in other words, that transplantation success did not depend only on the ability of the surgeon performing it. Up until Medawar's time, most surgeons thought that, if they could perform a technically perfect graft, the transplantation would work. Medawar showed that this was wrong: there was the fundamental barrier of compatibility to be overcome in order for skin grafts between genetically different people to work, because transplanted cells or tissues are recognized as non-self by the human immune system. This moved us onto the right path for making transplantation the life-saving medical reality it is today.

In the 1950s, however, Medawar would often deny that his research had any direct medical implications because his research didn't reveal a method for human transplantation.[1] His way of circumventing the natural barrier to transplantation had been shown to work only with young animals, and he was cautious about claiming too much medical significance for his basic research. Medawar probably wouldn't have agreed with James Watson's characteristic statement that you need to over-promise to be successful.[2]

It wasn't until the 1960s that Medawar became less cautious about transplantation working for humans.[3] Today, genetic matching between people and the use of immune-suppressive drugs make clinical transplantation a life-saving reality – directly building upon Medawar's insights. Such success in human transplantation has altered our very perception of what constitutes life and death.

In fact, the point at which death can be said to have taken place has itself become ambiguous. It used to be that, to determine life, people checked for a pulse or simply listened for someone's breathing. Now, the situation is far more complex: mechanical ventilators, pacemakers and drugs are able to sustain the circulation of air or blood in somebody who would otherwise die.

In 1968, an ad hoc committee assembled at Harvard Medical School to establish explicit criteria for death.[4] The committee had an all-star cast. It was chaired by Henry Beecher from Harvard Medical School, already renowned for being a whistle blower on human experimentation happening frequently without the patient's permission and for being the first to take account of the placebo effect in analysing clinical trials. The committee also included Joseph Murray, who had performed the first kidney transplantation between living people in December 1954,[5] and experts in neurosurgery, law, psychiatry and theology. The committee's work was urgent because public attention had been focused on the problem of defining death following the first heart transplant, performed a few months earlier, in December 1967, in Cape Town, South Africa, by forty-five-year-old surgeon Christiaan Barnard. The heart transplantation was deemed a success, even though the patient, fifty-five-year-old Louis Washkansky, would die eighteen days later from pneumonia.

Washkansky is the less-remembered hero of the world's first heart transplant story. As well as heart problems, Washkansky, a grocer, had diabetes and liver- and kidney-failure, and it was, perhaps, inevitable that, for a process still in its pioneering stage with many unknowns, the first heart transplant patient would have to be very near death. Washkansky, though, was a hero not – or not only – because he didn't hesitate to undergo an operation that had never before been performed successfully. Indeed, by this stage, anything was worth a shot for him. Rather, he was extraordinary for hanging on long enough to get his chance at life.

Along with Barnard and Washkansky there was a third hero to this medical first – Edward Darvall, the father who gave permission for his daughter's heart to be used in the experiment. Washkansky had been waiting for a suitable donor for three weeks when an ambulance arrived with Denise Darvall, a twenty-five-year-old girl who had just been run over by a drunk driver after getting out from her family car to buy a cake. Her mother had also been hit and she was already dead. Denise arrived in hospital with a broken leg, pelvis and skull, and severe brain damage – but an uninjured heart. Unimaginably distraught, her father was asked to decide whether or not Barnard could take his daughter's heart. He spent four minutes weighing his choices. He remembered how his daughter was always giving away things to other people. So surely, he thought to himself, she would have said yes.[6]

With that, Barnard moved a young girl's heart into an older man. But not before he was unexpectedly overwhelmed with doubt. He prayed while taking a shower before the operation: 'Oh Lord, please guide my hands tonight.'[7] One moment in particular sheds light on the state of mind of Barnard and his team. Darvall was already declared dead, and it was in Washkansky's best interest for the team to get the heart out while it was beating, minimizing the risk of it becoming damaged. But instead of doing what was medically best, they waited for Darvall's heart to stop beating entirely. They couldn't bring themselves to actually remove a still-beating heart. That would be a fraction too close to playing God.

At 6:13 a.m. on 3 December 1967, after an operation lasting four and a half hours, Darvall's heart began beating in Washkansky. Barnard later wrote that 'from birth [my life] had built towards one moment in an operating theatre when a blue heart turned red with life and a man was reborn. At that moment two lives had been fused into one.'[8] The grandiosity of Barnard's sentiment was deserved; his transplant success was momentous. Kidney transplantation had been achieved many years earlier but the public were captivated by the transfer of the most symbolic organ of all, the heart. After all, nobody writes poems about kidneys.

Immediately after the transplantation, Barnard became a celebrity. 'On Saturday, I was a surgeon in South Africa, very little known. On Monday I was world-renowned.' And two years later he divorced his wife. He embarked on a string of relationships with glamorous and famous women, marrying twice more – the third time, when in his *actually 2440 -*

mid-sixties, to an eighteen-year-old model. He became outspoken on a range of issues, from protesting against South African apartheid to suggesting that Princess Diana could have survived her 1997 car-crash had the emergency services in Paris acted differently.

Many surgeons around the world had raced to perform the first successful heart transplantation, and nobody suspected Barnard would be first. In the same week as Barnard's operation, a Brooklyn hospital tried and failed to give a new heart to a nineteen-day-old child.[9] In London, meanwhile, a physician attempted to persuade the National Heart Hospital to attempt a heart transplant but, according to the physician, the hospital delayed the operation because of complex ethical and legal problems and the patient died waiting.[10] It was perhaps inevitable that the first successful heart transplant would take place in a country with less red tape, because the ethical and legal problems were so intractable.

To transplant a heart, it has to be fresh. But how could anyone take a beating heart out of somebody when to do so would kill them? The answer required establishing the concept of 'brain death' or 'irreversible coma' – and this was precisely the term used by the committee assembled at Harvard in 1968, to deal with the problem that Barnard's successful transplant had made prescient.

The committee deliberated from January to August 1968 before agreeing on four criteria as defining this new state of human existence. The patient's body had to manifest: 1) no response to pain, 2) no spontaneous movement, 3) no reflexes, and 4) no electrical activity in the brain.[11] These conditions had to persist for at least twenty-four hours, in the absence of any nervous-system depressants. Behind these criteria lies the subtle idea that not all our tissues and cells die at the same time. So someone's nervous system can be dead – and the person is truly unable to function in any way – but other organs could still be 'alive', able to work fine for a while longer. This was already agreed in the medical profession – albeit unofficially – and probably the biggest impact of the Harvard Committee's report was to propel the issue of brain death to the forefront of public and academic scrutiny.

Philosophical, ethical, legislative and religious literature erupted in response. Just three months after Barnard's success, US Senator Walter Mondale opened a subcommittee hearing on the questions raised by transplantation and said: 'These advances and others yet to come raise grave and fundamental ethical and legal questions for our society – who shall live and who shall die; how long shall life be preserved and how shall it be altered; who shall make decisions; how shall society be prepared.'[12] Popular magazines *Reader's Digest* and *Time* also discussed the issues and questioned whether it was appropriate for a doctor to unilaterally decide when death occurs – where do the family's wishes fit in?[13]

On the other hand, some medical professionals felt the criteria were already too restrictive and proposed, in the mid-1970s, that brain death be defined by a loss of higher-brain functions, rather than requiring all electrical signals in the brain to be inactive. When the brain loses its higher functions, so the argument ran, psychological traits of that person are lost: death, in other words, has really occurred. It's easy to see from here how defining brain death is highly problematic. Compounding the difficulties, patients fulfilling the criteria for brain death may not appear dead. They might still be breathing, even if being helped to do so artificially. There is trauma for everyone involved in this ultimate decision.

In making such judgements, people often look to religion for guidance. Considerable resistance to designating somebody as 'brain dead' when seeking transplant donors has come, for example, from some branches of Orthodox Judaism, which insist that an irreversible end to cardiac and respiratory activity must remain the only criterion for death. Other branches of Judaism – Conservative and Reform Judaism, for instance – have been more accommodating. As far as the Catholic Church is concerned, Pope Pius XII paved the way forward in 1957 when he clarified that responsibility for giving a clear and precise definition of death lay with the doctor. For Islam, the Qur'an itself does not precisely define death, but some Islamic countries, such as Turkey, now have explicit laws that accept the definition of brain death. Hinduism, Protestantism and many other world religions similarly do not have any formal resistance to the idea of brain death.[14]

Still, the debate will only ever become more difficult as new medical advances will inevitably complicate the situation further. Brain parts cannot be transplanted today, but what if this were to become possible in the future? Such an idea may seem monstrous, but in the late

1960s many claimed it was monstrous to transplant a heart. While we have long since stopped considering the heart as the body's emotional, soulful core, higher-brain function really could contain something of our identity. Rather than a robust and all-encompassing philosophical definition of death that can endure through future medical advances, we have more of a practical consensus amongst medical practitioners that works within current technology.[15]

Today, someone certified as brain dead can pass on their heart, lungs, liver, kidneys, pancreas, intestine and tissues, including corneas, skin and bone. One donor can save or transform the lives of up to nine others. Nevertheless, every day, three people in the UK and seventy-seven in the US die while waiting for the right donor.[16] As Medawar made us realize back in the 1950s, the problem is the immune reaction against somebody else's tissues and cells. If the right match can be made between donor and recipient, this obstacle can be overcome. But

people? What a

ferent people –

Long before

thing at all abo

reactions was

of different ty

carry oxygen,

ecules include

primary issue

that different

names of the w

fact that some

AB), while oth

The Austria

groups in 1901

hadn't had an e

medical doctor

after spending

1897 only on a

at Trieste was t

a paid research

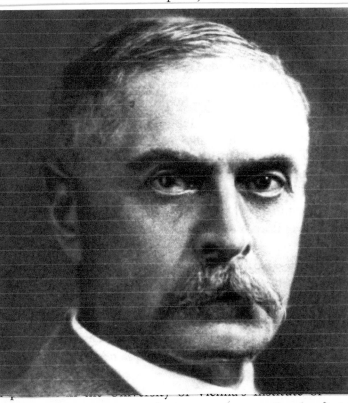

Karl Landsteiner

Pathological Anatomy – officially as an assistant to the institute's head, although in practice he pursued his own ideas.[17] Not until after his discovery of blood groups would he become a full member of the University's medical faculty.

Having read about experiments showing that human blood can react to animal blood, Landsteiner wondered if a reaction might occur when blood from different people was mixed together. He reasoned that, since blood from different species must vary, perhaps blood from individuals within the same species also differs. In 1901, he set about testing this with a characteristically simple – yet rigorous and brilliant – experiment. He began by taking blood from six women who had recently given birth – perhaps because these samples were easy to obtain – and separated their red blood cells from the serum (the liquid part of blood, without cells or clotting factors). He then mixed cells from one person with the serum from another, in all possible combinations, and drew up a table detailing whether or not a reaction – indicated by the red blood cells clumping together – occurred in each instance.

He couldn't explain what caused the cells to clump (we now know that it's part of a specific immune response) but he looked for patterns in whose cells and serum reacted. Nobody's serum reacted when recombined with their own cells. But cells combined with serum from different people did react in some cases. According to the predominant view of the time, which held that problems with blood transfusions reflected one's history of disease, this reaction might have been ascribed to the presence of disease within some of the samples that caused cells from others to clump.[18] Landsteiner, however, had an epiphany. What if, he thought, his results indicated not disease, but simply a natural incompatibility between different people's blood?

Immediately, he next tried the same experiment with six people from his own research lab, including himself. The importance of this second experiment was that he knew these people weren't ill in any obvious way and so any reactions seen this time would be unlikely to be caused by disease. He again found that some people's cells and serum would react. He became confident that his hunch was right – that there was a natural variation in different people's blood. But was there any pattern to the reactions? It was a huge leap forward for science when he realized that he could account for the pattern of reactions by proposing that humans have three different types of blood – he called them A, B and C (C being what we now call O, the blood type that lacks both A and B sugars).

At first, not even Landsteiner – never mind anybody else – quite realized how supremely important this discovery was. When reporting these experiments in his paper 'Agglutination of normal people's blood', published in German in 1901, he concluded by saying: 'I hope this will be of some use.'[19] Landsteiner always spoke humbly of his achievements. Even as late as 1930, in a very rare public interview that he gave to the Austrian daily newspaper *Der Wiener Tag* soon after the announcement that these experiments had won him the Nobel Prize, he said that his discovery of blood groups would surely not interest a layperson.[20] Of course, the truth is that this is of immense importance to us – it paved the way for successful blood transfusions, and, fundamentally, these experiments revealed the first molecular mark of our individual differences.

Medawar would later call Landsteiner's work one of the great triumphs of modern clinical biology.[21] But at the time it took many years for Landsteiner's discoveries to become widely known; he wasn't one for actively seeking to promote his work and he made no effort to make his papers easy to read – telling the truth was all he aspired to in his writing.[22] It wasn't until doctors had to explain why their blood transfusions often didn't work at the start of the First World War that the enormity of Landsteiner's discovery became widely recognized. Even then, long after the practical importance of his work was clear, a letter that Landsteiner wrote to his student on 12 February 1921 indicates he was being criticized by some scientists in the US because his original paper in 1901 only described three blood groups, whereas, in fact, there are four.[23] It had simply taken another year for the fourth, much rarer, group (AB) to be identified by one of Landsteiner's students.[24]

Science meant everything to Landsteiner, and he worked long hours for these experiments while living in seclusion with his mother, with whom he had a close relationship following his father's death, when Landsteiner was aged seven. He lived with his mother until her death in April 1908, by which time Landsteiner was aged forty-nine, and it was only at this point that he married. He kept a cast of his mother's face on his bedroom wall for the rest of his life. In the lab, he was a good mentor to some but he also soured relationships with others by complaining often about his working conditions. He found long-term friendships difficult.[25]

When going to Stockholm in 1930 to collect his Nobel Prize, it's curious that he didn't take his wife or son with him. In fact, when he heard that he had won the prize he didn't even tell his wife or son about it at first – they only found out later that evening when a friend came round to visit.[26] Also strange is that in the group photos of the 1930 Nobel Prize winners, everyone is facing the front except for Landsteiner – he turned his chair to face sideways, deliberately looking in a different direction to everyone else around him. Landsteiner, it can safely be said, was nothing if not eccentric.

At the turn of the twentieth century, around the time that Landsteiner discovered blood groups, the work of another Austrian burst into view – even though this Austrian was long dead. The Austrian monk Gregor Mendel had died in 1884, aged sixty-one, with his lifetime's work remaining unknown – his seminal discovery, written in 1865, was published in forty-four pages entitled 'Experiments on plant hybrids' in the journal of the local Brünn Biological Society. On 8 May 1900, the British zoologist William Bateson took a train from Cambridge to London. With him, he had Mendel's seminal paper, which had been published thirty-five years earlier. Mendel had spent his time in his monastery's greenhouse, cross-pollinating pea plants to know how peas' colour and shape passed from one generation to the next. He discovered wrinkled and smooth pea plants, for example, didn't blend this trait to produce offspring with just slightly wrinkled peas. Rather, the next generation were either smooth or wrinkled, just like one of the parents. The huge importance of this horticultural observation was that it implied that traits are inherited in discrete units; which we now call genes.

Mendel's paper had been recently cited by Dutch and German scientists and, as his train steamed along, Bateson settled back in his seat and was instantly gripped.[27] According to recollections of Bateson's wife, Beatrice, he quickly realized the impact of Mendel's work – that traits must be inherited in discrete units – and henceforth championed the discovery. In 1905, he coined the term 'genetics' and so began a new branch of science.

Like everyone at the time, Landsteiner was not aware of Mendel's work until Bateson and others rediscovered it. So Landsteiner had not initially considered that blood groups could be inherited but when he did, probably one or two years after Bateson's train ride, he immediately realized that blood groups could help out in paternity disputes,[28] which was in effect an early use of the power of genetic fingerprinting. We now know that your blood group is determined by a gene involved in adding sugar molecules to the surface of red blood cells. This gene comes in A, B and O forms. So, if you inherited the A version of this gene from your mother and the B version from your father, then your red blood cells will have both A and B sugars and you'll be blood group AB; inherit two A genes and you'll be blood group A, and so on.

As a foetus, your immune system learns to be tolerant to your own blood-group sugars. This, of course, is Burnet's and Medawar's theory of acquired tolerance in action. But your blood serum contains antibodies able to attack the versions of those sugars that you don't possess. Somebody who's blood group A cannot, for example, accept blood from a B group donor because a huge immune reaction will occur which can cause fever, shock, kidney failure, and may be even be fatal.[29]

Showing the foresight of a truly great scientist, Landsteiner even tried to relate his discoveries in blood group compatibility to problems in skin grafting.[30] But this had to wait for Medawar and Burnet. While working in his lab, Landsteiner suffered a heart attack on 24 June 1943 and reluctantly went to hospital, where he died two days later. Every scientist dies with the frustration of problems being unsolved.

Blood-group genes come in just three versions – such human differences are simple compared to the immense variation in our compatibility genes that control skin graft success. Recall that these genes vary *the most* from person to person. There are three compatibility genes that encode for proteins found on nearly all cells in your body (formally called *class I* compatibility genes) and these are termed A, B and C. You inherit a set of these three genes from your mother and another from your father. In this way, we each have six different class I compatibility genes: 2 As, 2 Bs and 2 Cs. It's theoretically possible to inherit several identical genes from Mum and Dad, but that's unlikely, because in all there are 1,243 versions of the A gene, 1,737 different B genes and 884 Cs found so far.[31] So the number of combinations in these genes that we can each inherit is mind-boggling.

In Landsteiner's experiments mixing serums with red blood cells, compatibility genes weren't important. That's because human red blood cells are short-lived cells with the relatively straightforward task of carrying oxygen around the body and – unlike most human cells – they don't have the proteins encoded by compatibility genes.[32] But matching compatibility genes is the major factor for the long-term success of organ transplants.

For most organ transplants, hospitals will assess the match between recipient and potential donors across two class I compatibility genes – A and B – and one of the class II compatibility genes called DR. If a perfect match isn't available, they will check directly whether or not the recipient has an acute immune reactivity against the donor's cells. For bone marrow transplants, they also check the match of two other compatibility genes, C and DQ.[33] For a kidney transplant in which no genes were matched, the half-life of the graft would be about seven years – but if the most important six can be matched, the graft's half-life rises to between twelve and twenty years. This is, of course, fantastic, but it also leads to dilemmas.

While prioritizing matched compatibility genes improves the outcome of transplantation, it also leads to a racial imbalance in who receives a transplant. This is because some variants of our compatibility genes are more prevalent in certain groups of people. Indeed, analysis of transplantation and survival rates across the US suggested that, if we ignored trying to match the B compatibility gene, there would be a small increase in the rate of transplantation failure but also an increase in the number of ethnically non-white people in the US finding a suitable match.[34] This is just one example of a tension inherent in establishing transplantation priority.

So how did we uncover the extraordinary variation in compatibility genes among the human population? In fact, this was discovered in the same way Landsteiner discovered blood groups – by serology – that is, by testing how serum from one person reacts with cells from someone else. Three research teams opened up this frontier of human biology, presenting their key discoveries about human compatibility, in the late 1950s and early 1960s.[35]

First, forty-two-year-old Jean Dausset, working in Paris, reported that serum from people who had previously had several blood transfusions would react with some other people's white blood cells, causing them to clump. This was very similar to what Landsteiner observed when studying red blood cell reactions, the difference here being that Dausset observed an effect with white blood cells using serum taken from people who had previously had blood transfusions. The blood transfusion had triggered an immune response against the donor's white cells, leaving the patient poised to react again to cells that carried the same non-self protein. Such a reaction would be dangerous, potentially lethal, if it occurred after a blood transfusion – because the immune system would go into overdrive, attacking cells in the transfused blood.

In 1958, Dausset didn't know what was causing the reaction; all he knew was that one person's serum could react with another person's white blood cells. So he named what was being recognized as MAC, because three key volunteers in his experiments had names beginning with M, A and C. Indeed, Dausset took great care to pay tribute to the volunteers used in his research. He noted that the 'only truly remarkable and deeply inspiring aspect of this adventure' was the large number of volunteers offering themselves to serve humanity.[36]

In parallel with Dausset, Rose Payne at Stanford, California, then in her late forties, and Jon van Rood in Leiden, Holland, then in his early thirties, each independently made another observation caused by our variation in compatibility genes. They found that serum from mothers with several children could cause other people's white blood cells to clump together – indicating an immune reaction. Van Rood – who wrote up his findings in his 1962 PhD thesis – was struck by one particular patient who reacted very badly to a single blood transfusion. A mother of four had given birth to twins and, because of significant bleeding, she was given her first-ever blood transfusion. But she reacted badly, started shaking and collapsed.[37] Normally, reactions like this only occurred after several blood transfusions. It was known that patients could be sensitized to non-self proteins in one blood transfusion so that a bad reaction occurs when the immune system sees the same non-self proteins in a further transfusion. But why would this woman react so badly to her first-ever blood transfusion?

Seeing patients react to their first transfusion led van Rood, as well as Payne in Stanford, to wonder if these people had been already sensitized for an immune reaction in some way other than a previous transfusion. Looking at the medical records, van Rood wondered if the woman who collapsed could have been sensitized to non-self proteins during her previous pregnancies – those from the baby's father.[38] His hunch was proved right when he demonstrated that blood taken from women with several children often did react strongly to other people's white blood cells (causing the cells to clump together). This implied that mothers can be exposed to blood or cells from the baby – most likely during the birth, when there's often a lot of tissue damage – and as a result, they become sensitized to the father's proteins.

The work of these three independent researchers – reporting these related phenomena – amounts to nothing less than the discovery of a new-found human variability. As distinct in its own way as skin, hair or eye colour, this variation is hidden deep within us, only revealed when blood parts from different people were mixed together.

Yet this new-found human characteristic is far more variable than skin, hair or eye colour. And the enormous range in human compatibility genes – the underlying cause of the reactions observed by Dausset, Payne and van Rood – made their observations very difficult to analyse, compared to Landsteiner's simple blood groups. As Dausset tried to find patterns in the data, his laboratory was slowly transformed, plastered in posters with pluses, minuses and ranked scales of reaction intensities, between different cells and sera.[39]

The most frustrating outcome of any experiment is when the results don't seem to show a clear pattern; and Dausset simply couldn't see any logic behind the array of data on his walls. Payne's and van Rood's data on mothers were easier to analyse, because the mothers' sera was sensitized to the baby's father while blood transfusion patients, on the other hand, had been exposed to blood from multiple donors, making the sera's reactivity more complex. Dausset realized this and set up a series of transfusions using blood from one single donor to make things simpler.

Payne also understood that improvements in statistical analysis would be invaluable in revealing the patterns of reactivity. Help came in the form of the Briton Walter Bodmer, the son of a Jewish doctor who had always wanted one of his children to go into medicine.[40] Bodmer had recently obtained his PhD at Cambridge University, working with a pioneer in modern statistics, Ronald Fisher, and arrived in Stanford in the summer of 1961 on a one-year fellowship to work with Josh Lederberg – the same Josh Lederberg who had earlier taught Nossal in Australia how to use the micromanipulator, which allowed Nossal to isolate immune cells and prove each one could neutralize only one type of bacteria.

On Thursday, 15 February 1962, Bodmer heard Payne give a talk about her research on the newly found human variability, and from that Bodmer worked, together with his wife Julia, on statistical analyses of Payne's data. From that time on, the Bodmers played a leading role in deciphering the compatibility gene system, and their early simple statistical tests proved to be crucial in working out what was going on – helped by the novelty of using computers for medical research.[41] Bodmer's one-year fellowship turned into a nine-year-long stay in Stanford.[42]

Even with statistical analysis, it was soon clear that no lab in the world had enough samples or resources on their own to resolve the complexities of compatibility genes. While Medawar and Burnet met relatively rarely and could happily exchange ideas through each other's published papers, this was an entirely different situation; the new band of pioneers had to meet so they could directly swap and compare cells and sera. They established a series of international meetings attended by everyone in the world studying the compatibility gene system – initially about fourteen teams in all. This was a ground-breaking level of international cooperation, the forerunner of collaborations in the Human Genome Project or the Large Hadron Collider. As a result, our understanding of the compatibility genes was completely transformed. In the early 1960s, the sense of what they were was still haphazard; by the end of the decade, it had come into clear focus – largely because of the series of international meetings that the different research groups gathered at.

Still, the first of these meetings – in 1964, at Duke University, North Carolina, organized by Bernard Amos, another of the early pioneers in compatibility genes – was a disaster. At the meeting it became clear that the different techniques each lab used gave discordant results. Tests using the exact same cells and sera gave different results merely depending on who did it. In one tense moment at the meeting, the highly respected leading Italian geneticist Ruggero Ceppellini said Dausset's data was worthless, literally ripping up Dausset's datasheets.[43] Optimism waned, and everyone dispersed to troubleshoot their methods.

Van Rood, ever a hard-working and popular leader, organized a second get-together the following year in Leiden, Holland.[44] And this time, things went much better.[45] MAC, named by Dausset, turned out to be identical to what was being recognized in sera being used by at least four other groups, each of whom had given it different names such as LA2 (Payne and Bodmer) or 8a (van Rood).[46] Many other patterns of reactivity emerged, and the extent of this new-found human diversity began to be seen more clearly.[47]

In 1967, the World Health Organization (WHO) established a committee to determine an official naming system for the relevant genes.[48] Establishing a nomenclature wasn't just a matter of semantics: naming things required everyone to agree on how to organize the information, which in turn required working out the underlying principles. It was the beginning of bringing order to the data. As Bodmer put it, 'nomenclature is the biologist's closest equivalent to the mathematician's notation'.[49]

A recording of the first meeting focused on naming compatibility genes, in New York in 1968, preserves the enthusiasm of the thirteen attendees, but also reveals the uncertainties of the time. 'I agree with you [but] we should define what we are talking about,' was the kind of blunt, honest banter that ricocheted around that meeting. 'We're digressing. We're not sticking to the points. Are you sticking to the points?' Everything was questioned – often coarsely. A comment from Bodmer summarizes the essence of the problem: 'The devil is that ... you don't really know what you're dealing with. You don't know whether you're dealing with one system, with a hundred systems, with one basic chemical substance modified by many enzymes controlled by a set of closely linked systems or what.'[50]

Still, that first meeting in New York set in motion the nomenclature for compatibility genes that's in use today. The committee still exists and sets the official names for any newly discovered variants of these genes. Early on, however, a problem was apparent. The issue stemmed from the fact that there were two types of test that could be done with a person's white blood cells. In one, the reactivity of blood serum to another person's white blood cells was tested, and in the other kind of test, different people's white blood cells were mixed together – which would also sometimes react. In both cases, a reaction triggered the cells to change shape and start multiplying. The problem was that, to everyone's surprise, reactivity between sera and cells was not always predictive of the mixed cell reactions. How could this be?

One possible explanation was that there were different kinds of compatibility genes, each being revealed in the different types of test. At first, nobody understood how this could be, but nevertheless compatibility genes were divided into two groups, class I and class II, according to whether they were identified by reactions between serum and cells (class I) or by reactions in mixtures of white blood cells (class II). Eventually it was discovered that class I proteins were indeed found on nearly all types of cells, but class II proteins were only found on some types of immune cells – and that led to these discordant results.

The human compatibility genes were named as the HLA (human leukocyte antigen) genes. We now know that there are three class I HLA genes, denoted as A, B and C. Each human being also has three sets of class II genes, called HLA-DR, -DP and -DQ.[51] The versions of these genes that you can inherit are each very similar, but the differences have been carefully catalogued. Each version of these genes, both class I and class II, has been assigned a number by the WHO committee. So, for example, each possible version of A, B and C gene has been assigned a number: one person may have, for example, genes A*02 and A*11 (said simply as A-two and A-eleven), meaning that they have two particular variants of the A gene.[52] Some variants are very rare, others quite common. For example, well over a quarter of the population of England have A*02 – formally said as human leukocyte antigen A*02, or HLA-A*02 – and a similar frequency is found in European Americans, whereas only about 6 per cent have HLA-A*11. Indeed, A*02 is particularly common worldwide, but the frequency of most

57

versions of these genes varies a lot in different populations: A*11, for instance, is about five times more common among Singapore Chinese than in England. MAC, discovered by Dausset, is the version of the A gene now named HLA-A*02 and it was detected first because it's a globally common version of HLA-A.

Dausset won the Nobel Prize in 1980. It was, however, a close community – rather than one individual – assembled in this string of international meetings, that opened up this new research field. 'What a unique privilege for me,' Dausset said in 1990, 'in friendly association with the other pioneers, to have lived through the exalting and rebounding episodes of this great adventure.'[53] Everyone knew everyone else very well. Still, this small band of pioneers had struck gold, and there was inevitably game-playing by some trying to emphasize their primacy in the field. It's perhaps not surprising that recollections vary somewhat between the major players in the early days of HLA regarding who contributed what and when exactly.[54] Many consider van Rood to have been very unlucky to have been left out of the 1980 Nobel Prize.[55]

As discoveries in HLA moved along, the practical impact on transplantation also moved along. Dausset converted his administrative office into an operating room for studying skin-graft reactions.[56] He performed small skin grafts on the forearms of volunteers and tried to correlate the results with HLA types.[57] In the mid-1960s Paul Terasaki at UCLA, who previously worked with Peter Medawar in London,[58] proposed a clinical trial for the importance of matching HLA when using organs from post-mortem donors (cadavers), and van Rood proposed the first international organ exchange programme.[59] By the early 1970s, it was clear that success in kidney transplantation was hugely favoured between HLA-matched siblings.[60]

We now know that the degree to which our compatibility genes control transplantation success generally depends on what is being transplanted. For liver transplants, for example, matching HLA types between donor and recipient is not as important as it is in transplantation of other organs. It's not entirely clear why, but it's probably down to two special things about the liver: firstly, the liver is very good at regenerating – and hence healing – itself; and secondly, interestingly, the liver is a part of our body relatively protected from immune reactions.

The liver receives blood from the intestine, which contains products from food we eat, and the bacteria that live in our gut. So the liver is continuously exposed to non-self. But this non-self isn't harmful; you don't want food or normal gut bacteria to trigger an immune reaction. It's not entirely understood how the immune system is prevented from reacting against harmless non-self molecules in the liver, but it is known, for example, that particular secretions from liver cells inhibit immune reactions. Of course, limiting immune responses in the liver makes it a convenient place for germs to hide, and indeed infection of the liver with the hepatitis B virus leads to around a million deaths a year worldwide.[61]

Some other places in our body are protected from immune reactions for a different reason; parts of us are just too important to become a battle zone. When immune cells kill diseased cells, healthy cells in the area can be inadvertently killed and affected by debris from destroyed cells or secretions from the immune cells. Put simply, an immune response is destructive wherever it occurs. Some tissues or cells may be so important that it is best to take a chance with the presence of germs there, rather than risking an immune response there. Privileged parts of us, too precious for an immune response to occur easily, include our eyes, brain, and – for half of us – our testes.

For a long time, there has been the hope that insight into how immune responses are kept under control in such organs would lead to new ideas for helping transplantation work. But we still haven't mastered how the immune system becomes more tolerant in these organs. Transplantation triggered the revolution in our understanding of the immune system – but immunology is yet to pay back its debt and solve the problem of transplantation in return.

While not solving the problem fully, our understanding of immune responses helps transplant patients in the application of matching compatibility genes between donors and recipients, and in the use of immune-suppressive drugs, which are the mainstay of post-transplant treatment.[62] Drugs like azathioprine, which stops immune cells multiplying, allowed the first kidney transplants to be done in the 1960s; cyclosporine, which similarly stops immune cell activation, first isolated from a fungus found in soil in 1969, caused a step-change in survival curves from the 1980s onwards. And there's another, surprising, benefit from our understanding of immune responses in transplant patients. It comes from the discovery that immune reactions can occur both ways between donor and recipient; not only can the patient's immune system kill the transplant, but immune cells in the transplant itself can attack the patient – for example, in bone-marrow transplants, when the transplant contains many of the donor's immune cells. An attack by immune cells within the transplant causes so-called graft-versus-host disease, which needs treatment with immune-suppressive drugs.

Yet, surprisingly, such disease can have its benefits. A bone-marrow transplant to treat leukaemia or myeloma not only aims to replace cancerous cells with healthy cells, but also provides new immune cells from the donor, which can then attack any remaining cancer cells in the recipient. One key problem, then, lies in taking measures to prevent graft-versus-host disease while still giving grafted immune cells a chance to help attack cancerous cells.

More exotic routes to improving clinical transplantation have also been explored. Organs from animals have been considered as a way of solving problems with donor shortage.[63] But this raises many difficulties. First is the issue of whether or not animal physiology is close enough to human for transplanted tissues or organs to work properly. And then there's the immune problem: animal cells are clearly going to be seen as non-self. Pigs have been considered suitable donors for some tissues, but pig cells contain a particular sugar molecule, also found on bacteria, that is not found in humans. As a way round that problem, pig cells have been engineered to lack that particular sugar, but something else on pig cells still triggered an immune response. For now, pretty much the only way animal parts end up in humans is by us eating them – but there are exceptions, such as the common practice of replacing human heart valves with pig ones.

With the benefit of hindsight, knowing that transplantation can work and that genetic matching is so important, it is fascinating that, in fact, the discovery of HLA was not a watershed moment for most scientists at the time. The pioneers – Dausset, van Rood, Payne and the teams who swapped cells and ideas in the series of meetings which began at Duke University in 1964 – had the field to themselves for many years before others recognized its importance.

The reason it took a while for others to catch on was that enormous variation in human compatibility genes didn't immediately provide a new concept about the nature of humanity. Without a full knowledge of what these do, it took a leap of faith to think they were important. Quite simply, nobody knew at first why these genes were so different between people. Everyone agreed that these genes couldn't exist just to make transplantation difficult. So what is the true role of our compatibility genes? The answer required a different era of biological science, in which molecular and cellular details drive progress. And only then, through the work of a different group of scientists digging deep into how our immune system works, do we finally gain a clear picture of what compatibility genes really do.

4

A Crystal-clear Answer at Last

On 15 November 2001, the American microbiologist Don Wiley disappeared into thin air. His car was found near Memphis, on the Hernando De Soto Bridge, which spans the Mississippi river, unlocked, with its keys still in the ignition. For weeks, the Memphis police scoured the area and found nothing. It was only two months after the 9/11 attacks, and the FBI was called in to investigate, because Wiley was one of the world's leading authorities on dangerous viruses – he was familiar with HIV, Ebola, smallpox, herpes and influenza – and his disappearance was very strange. The fact that his wife and kids had just arrived in Memphis for a holiday they had all looked forward to hinted that it wasn't suicide. And, unlike many bridge jumpers, Wiley hadn't taken his shoes off first.

He had last been seen earlier that night, at a banquet for the Scientific Advisory Board of St Jude Children's Hospital in Memphis. Peter Doherty, the renowned Australian immunologist and Nobel laureate, recalled that Wiley had been in good spirits.[1] The chairwoman of the board, Patricia Donahoe from Massachusetts General Hospital in Boston, told the *New York Times* that she 'certainly saw no signs of depression' on Wiley's part, adding that she was 'very suspicious that there was some form of accident or foul play'.[2] Harvard and St Jude Hospital offered a $10,000 reward for information as to what had happened.[3]

Wiley was a candidate for a Nobel Prize for his work with Jack Strominger and Pamela Bjorkman at Harvard during the 1980s.[4] Like the trinity of Billingham, Brent and Medawar before them, this trio changed for ever how we think about the immune system. Bjorkman, Strominger and Wiley worked together for one thing: to get a picture of the HLA protein made by compatibility genes, to see what it really looked like. In 1987, after eight years of research, they obtained a portrait of HLA-A*02, the same HLA that Dausset had discovered and named MAC in 1958. He didn't know how it worked, but Bjorkman, Strominger and Wiley's image vividly revealed precisely how HLA works. It became an icon, instantly recognizable to any medical scientist or student in immunology.

Why is a picture of a protein so important? A gene is essentially an instruction that cells can use to make a particular protein; and proteins are long chains of atoms: mostly carbon, mixed with a few other elements like nitrogen, hydrogen and oxygen. These atoms connect together in a string but, crucially, for each individual protein the string folds up into a particular complex structure. We are interested in this structure, because that often explains what that particular protein does, and how it does it. An analogy is in how structural beams of a bridge are arranged to support a platform going from one side to another; simply the look of a bridge makes it clear what it does.

As the famous physicist Richard Feynman once quipped: 'It is very easy to answer many of these fundamental biological questions; you just look at the thing.'[5] The double-helix shape of DNA is a prototypical example of how the structures of biological molecules reveal how they work. The model of DNA built by Watson and Crick, in February 1953, showed that the components of DNA (the bases) linked in pairs across two helical strands. This meant that, if the strands separate, each can enable the addition of a new second strand, thereby making two copies of the double helix with the same sequence of bases. The celebrated structure of DNA is not ornament: it shows how DNA is able to copy itself, something central to our molecular understanding of heredity.[6] For understanding our immune system, the shape of the HLA protein – hard won by Bjorkman, Strominger and Wiley – was as revelatory as the DNA double helix.

At Harvard University in 1978, Pamela Bjorkman began her graduate studies aged twenty-two. Her parents, surprised at her having such a strong interest in science, thought it would be good for her to go to college so that she could meet a nice man there. Bjorkman herself said she felt like Harvard must have accepted her through some kind of clerical error, and her insecurity made her determined to prove her worth. Her destiny began to take shape when she heard Wiley give an inspiring talk at the department's autumn retreat at Woods Hole in Cape Cod.[7] Woods Hole, on the sea, worlds apart from the hubbub of Harvard, is a place where aspirations come easy. Wiley spoke about the structure of proteins, and his infectious, childlike enthusiasm hooked Bjorkman.

Stylish, tall and often dressed head-to-toe in black, Wiley was a rising star. After his PhD with the Nobel-Prize-winning chemist William Lipscomb, Wiley skipped several rungs of the usual career ladder, missing out years of lab work under somebody else's wing, to join Harvard's Department of Biochemistry and Molecular Biology in 1971. Despite this success, Wiley felt lost starting his own research lab so young – so much so that his motivation waned, and he thought of leaving science.[8] It wasn't that he lacked ideas; but the difficulty came from his burning desire to *only* work on something really important. Finding something he thought worthy enough to work on was the difficult part.

After three years at Harvard, in 1974, Wiley came up for promotion from an assistant to an associate professor, and Harvard hesitated, deciding to delay its decision for another two years in order to see whether or not his research programme was going to take off.[9] Eventually, Wiley found a worthy project: to determine the structure of influenza hemagglutinin, a protein that coats the 'flu virus and helps it stick to human cells. The outcome sealed his reputation for brilliance, as he discovered that the protein dramatically changes its shape to force an entrance for the 'flu virus to get inside our cells.

Wiley suggested to Bjorkman that she could continue with research on the influenza protein, but Bjorkman's friend Jim Kaufman – today a renowned scientist in Cambridge University but then working nearby in Jack Strominger's lab – told her that he couldn't think of anything more boring to work on, because the big discovery for that protein had already been made.[10] He suggested that instead she could try to get a structure of the HLA protein,[11] and so, in June 1979, Bjorkman began her work with Wiley and Strominger on HLA.

Strominger, by then aged fifty-four, had begun his career as an undergraduate at Harvard. He had been surprised at being accepted, because there were quotas in place to limit the number of Jewish students admitted. He majored in Psychology, which he often said later was great training for running a research team. He went to medical school at Yale and witnessed there, in 1946, the first patients in the US to be treated with penicillin, something that made a deep impression on him.[12] During the early 1950s, he had a brush with McCarthyism – because he owned books by Marx and Lenin that were actually reading material for a political science course he took while in medical school – before he was cleared and went on to work in the National Institutes of Health (NIH), which was small at that time. Like Wiley, Strominger demonstrated a precocious ability and, aged just twenty-six, he was given money and space to start his own research programme.

Strominger left the NIH because McCarthyism had left a bad taste in his mouth for government service. After briefly working in Europe, he went to Washington University in St Louis, Missouri, where he then made seminal discoveries about how penicillin works. Strominger, among others, successfully identified the way that bacteria made their cell walls, and as the process was unravelled, each step was tested for its sensitivity to penicillin. The very last step in the process was the key – penicillin works by interfering with bacterial protein needed to strengthen the cell wall, the final step in its construction. As a result of this discovery, Strominger was hot property. He moved to the University of Wisconsin, Madison, in 1964 and was then head-hunted back to Harvard, joining its faculty in 1968, the same year as Barnard's successful heart transplant, and, crucially, set up his lab in the same building as Wiley.

Arriving back at Harvard, Strominger, who had just turned forty, was ambitious to take on a big new research problem.[13] With his background in the chemistry of bacteria, he hadn't yet read anything by Burnet or Medawar, but it was a time when transplantation biology was in the air.[14] Everyone knew it was an important research field with many unsolved problems. Strominger needed a way into it, and his chance came in a flash of inspiration while he was at a meeting in Paris.[15]

One of the speakers, Allan Davies, from the Microbial Research Establishment at Porton, UK, gave a talk suggesting that differences in sugar molecules may underlie HLA compatibility – just like the basic blood groups that Landsteiner had discovered, but more complex. Strominger was listening, enthralled. For years, he'd worked on unusual sugars found in bacterial cell walls, so – he reasoned – he could apply his knowledge of sugar chemistry to attack the transplantation problem. HLA would be his new research priority.

Over the following few years, through the mid-to-late 1960s, Strominger found out that, in fact, Davies was wrong: sugars have nothing to do with our differences in HLA. But by then there was no turning back; his lab was focused on HLA, and his work on penicillin had wound down. During the decade before Bjorkman started working on HLA in 1979, Strominger's lab had purified the HLA protein, figured out its composition, identified which parts varied and isolated the DNA that encoded it. When they met in the stairwell of the Fairchild Building, where they worked, Wiley and Strominger discussed working together to get the structure of the HLA protein; a researcher in Strominger's team, Peter Parham, had worked at the project for a while.[16] But it wasn't until 1979 – with the trio of Bjorkman, Strominger and Wiley assembled – that work on the problem started in earnest.

Wiley actually thought at first that the project probably wouldn't work.[17] The problem was, as Wiley knew, HLA proteins have sugars (formally called carbohydrates) attached. Although the sugars aren't anything to do with the enormous variation in HLA that humans have, as Strominger had found out, sugars can vary somewhat in their composition. Wiley thought the presence of a sugar attached to HLA would create problems for them trying to identify the specific structure of an HLA protein – indeed, most protein structures solved at that time were ones that didn't have carbohydrates associated with them. So Wiley told Bjorkman that she could start the project with the proviso that, if it didn't look hopeful after a year, she should give up and do something else. Bjorkman accepted the condition and, as a joint graduate student between Wiley and Strominger, set out to find the structure of HLA protein.

Proteins are generally around 10 nanometres long – a million lined up would reach a centimetre – and each contains about 20,000 atoms. Since the 1950s, scientists have used X-ray crystallography to pinpoint the position of these atoms and reveal a protein's structure. The process requires first growing a crystal of pure protein. A beam of X-rays is fired at the crystal and then, by detecting the positions at which X-rays come out after passing through the crystal, the shape of the protein can be calculated.

The process to first get crystals of the protein involves adding the HLA protein to liquids containing varying concentrations of salt and other components in the hope that crystals form. It was mostly luck as to when Bjorkman would hit upon the right combination for crystals to form. She also needed to have the HLA protein in enough quantity for screening all the conditions in which crystals might grow.

Strominger's lab had already worked out a way to obtain reasonable amounts of the HLA protein.[18] For this, they used cells derived from a person living in an Indiana Amish community who had inherited the same A and B class I HLA proteins from each parent – so, unlike the usual level of variability, they just had one type of HLA-A and -B.[19] Bjorkman could cut the HLA proteins off from the surface of these cells (by adding an enzyme called papain) and then just had to separate the HLA-A from the -B protein, which was relatively easy (using a standard procedure called ion exchange chromatography). With this, Bjorkman obtained a pure HLA-A protein, which happened to be HLA-A*02 in this particular person. To everyone's surprise, the first time she tried to make crystals, it worked. These first crystals weren't good enough to obtain a structure from – the crystal needs to be of a certain size and quality for X-ray analysis – but nevertheless, it was a start. Then her luck ran out – she couldn't get the right quality of crystals to grow.

For seven years, Bjorkman was in the lab each day from around 10 a.m. right through until the early hours of the next morning.[20] Harvard had an atmosphere that made scientists feel like they wouldn't make it unless they gave it their all. But she was giving it her all, and still the crystals were too small and too rare. She began to accept that it might never work.[21] Persevering, she had the 'romantic and stupid idea that I'll either do this or I'll fail'.[22] She had managed to fathom some details about the symmetry of the protein, and how its constituent parts were broadly arranged. To the outside world this wasn't much, but when a big discovery doesn't happen, you take refuge in the small ones.

It at least helped Bjorkman that there wasn't such intense competition as there is in this kind of science today. The small, self-contained community of researchers in protein structures knew that Wiley was working on the structure of HLA protein and so, by and large, others left the problem alone. The pressure on Bjorkman was largely of her own volition.

Bjorkman switched from using X-ray sources at Harvard to more powerful beams that had become available in a type of particle accelerator being built around the world at that time. Each trip – often to one in Cornell near New York and later to another in Hamburg, Germany – was intense, because her experiments would take second place to the high-energy physicists' research, and from one moment to the next she could never tell when the X-ray beam for her experiment would be switched on or off. On one occasion, she spent five days waiting for a beam to come on for her experiment, being told the whole time it would be on again in about an hour. On another trip, the X-ray camera was broken and – since each crystal could only be exposed to the beam once – she lost a whole year's worth of samples when the camera didn't record the X-ray pattern.

There was no eureka moment, but, by combining snippets of data from many experiments, Bjorkman squeezed out some success and she solved 90 per cent of the structure. But the final 10 per cent was strange and elusive. A monumental discovery was concealed in this enigmatic 10 per cent of protein that Bjorkman couldn't fathom – but the secret would stay hidden for another year. To understand what happened next, we need to back up a bit in time, because a lot had occurred since the pioneers in HLA – Dausset, van Rood and Payne – had begun the quest that Bjorkman, Strominger and Wiley were about to shed light on.

In the mid-1970s, Rolf Zinkernagel, a medical doctor from Basel, Switzerland, and the Australian Peter Doherty carried out a series of experiments which revealed the real biological importance of the HLA proteins. Working together in the Australian city of Canberra, as part of Burnet's 'school of immunology', the pair's research would later be ubiquitously celebrated, detailed in every immunology textbook and would earn them a Nobel Prize.

Doherty had a PhD in Neuropathology from Edinburgh University and had been working in Canberra since the end of 1971 – well over a year before Rolf Zinkernagel arrived in January 1973. Zinkernagel, on the other hand, had struggled to get a job and only landed a place in Canberra through personal discussions he had with scientists visiting the institute where he worked in Europe.[23] He moved to Australia with his wife and two small children – then aged two and a half years and eleven months – only to find out that there was little room in the crowded lab where he was due to work. He was directed to share workspace with Doherty, a small decision that turned out to have huge ramifications.

Zinkernagel and Doherty worked together for the next two and a half years, and their names are forever linked by this relatively brief moment of spectacular achievement. In hindsight, Doherty considers it a big advantage to them that Australia was still somewhat remote from the scientific mainstream – despite the legacy of Burnet and others at the Hall Institute – giving them the space to think differently. At the time, although HLA proteins were important for their role in transplantation, nobody had any idea what their real function could be in the body. There was evidence available to indicate that immune responses were influenced by specific genes, but research had focused on immune responses to chemically synthesized molecules.[24] Zinkernagel and Doherty, interested in these studies, thought it important to study an immune response against a real danger, like a virus.

Doherty was studying mouse immune responses to Lymphocytic Choriomeningitis Virus (LCMV). This virus is especially interesting to immunologists, because it's the immune reaction to the virus that causes the problems, rather than the virus itself. Immune cells, activated by the virus, kill cells that are critical for maintaining the blood–brain barrier, something that can lead to acute brain swelling and death. Recall how some parts of the body need to be protected from immune responses: this is an example of why such protection is necessary – and what happens when it fails.

Bonding through their dedication, passion and a mutually appreciated dry humour,[25] Zinkernagel and Doherty started working together on LCMV day and night, seven days a week. 'The experience was truly intense,' Doherty later recalled. 'We were totally obsessed.'[26] Together they tested first whether immune cells (specifically T cells) taken from the cerebal spinal fluid of infected animals could kill cells that they deliberately infected with the virus.[27] They found that the better the immune cells were at killing, the greater was the severity of the disease in mice: as expected for the disease being caused by the immune response, rather than the virus directly. Then, in October 1973, came their big breakthrough experiment.

Inspired by previous studies showing that strains of mice differed in their susceptibility to diseases, they set out to compare the ability of the immune cells from one mouse strain to kill virus-infected cells taken from other strains.[28] A series of experiments using cells taken from mice with different genetic backgrounds yielded a sensational discovery: that the immune cells, killer T cells specifically, could not kill just any cell infected with the virus.[29] What the pair found was that killer T cells activated by the virus in one mouse strain were *only* able to detect the virus in other cells that had the same class I compatibility genes. The implication was that genes for transplant compatibility also control immune responses against a virus.

This discovery was dynamite, and Zinkernagel and Doherty knew it. The pair presented their work to Burnet, by now aged seventy-four, but surprisingly he didn't appreciate the results instantly.[30] Undaunted, Zinkernagel and Doherty decided they should get out and tell people about their work: Doherty gave twenty-two talks across the world in six weeks, and Zinkernagel gave many others throughout Europe.[31] In April 1974, they published their results in the top journal *Nature*.[32] Even so, many still thought their observation was just some spurious result – perhaps something strange arising from the methods or the particular virus they used.[33] The scientific community acknowledged that these genes couldn't simply exist just to make life difficult for transplant surgeons – but it was hard for scientists to change ingrained patterns of thought and see these genes as being able to control the immune response to a virus. Most scientists at the time thought that an immune cell would recognize a virus infection directly – without any restriction or influence from the type of cell infected. Doherty, in particular, never forgot the names of those who poured cold water on his work.[34]

It was some two years after Zinkernagel and Doherty's *Nature* paper was published – around the time it took other teams to publish their own versions of the experiment – before the scientific community broadly agreed on the importance of this work. Zinkernagel and

Doherty coined the term 'MHC restriction' to describe the idea that the detection of viruses is restricted to cells with appropriate MHC proteins. (To be clear, MHC refers to compatibility genes in all species, and HLA is the acronym for these genes in humans.) 'MHC restriction' remains in the everyday language of immunologists.

In 1975, Zinkernagel and Doherty discussed the implications of their extraordinary discovery in a short but seminal piece for the *Lancet*.[35] In it, they introduced a new idea. Over twenty-five years earlier, in 1949, Burnet had articulated the idea that the immune system works by telling apart self and non-self, distinguishing your own cells and tissues from anything else. Zinkernagel and Doherty's new idea was to suggest that, in fact, the immune system works through recognition of 'altered self'. A body's MHC proteins, they proposed, were 'altered' by the presence of a virus – and the body's immune system could then identify disease as 'altered self'. This was an important shift in thinking about how the immune system worked.

They went further: to suggest that their data could explain why there is such great diversity in our HLA proteins. At the time, in the mid-1970s, the dominant explanation for this diversity was that transplantation incompatibility could have evolved to prevent tumours spreading among us. Transmissible cancers are not known to occur in humans – but they have been found in a few animals. A transmissible venereal tumour in dogs, for example, is passed on during copulation and may have originated when dogs were first domesticated around 10,000 years ago.[36] Zinkernagel and Doherty, however, speculated that diversity in HLA might relate to how a population avoids viral infections.

Perhaps, their argument ran, it would be harder for a virus to evade our immune system if the process of detection varies. Or, put another way, they speculated that we might have evolved diversity in HLA so that we are stronger at fighting off viruses – as a population. The idea proved to be very insightful, especially because it wasn't clear to anyone how the MHC protein could really be 'altered' by the presence of a virus – that wasn't going to be revealed until Bjorkman, Wiley and Strominger finally worked out what was going on in that elusive 10 per cent of the HLA protein structure. But, at the time, Zinkernagel and Doherty emphasized that such details were not central

71

to their general arguments; like Burnet before them, they were concerned with establishing principles for how the immune system works.

Zinkernagel and Doherty won the Nobel Prize in 1996 – surprisingly a long twenty years after they actually worked together on these ground-breaking experiments and ideas. Did they know it was coming? 'Well, people told me I'd been nominated for the Nobel Prize,' Doherty recalled to me in 2011, 'but I don't know how they knew as it's all supposed to be secret.'[37]

Following Zinkernagel and Doherty, the big question was *how* MHC proteins and viruses were being recognized together. What exactly – as in what protein or combination of proteins – could immune cells detect? This needed to be answered to understand how detection of a virus is linked to proteins encoded by our compatibility genes. A clear picture of how this works was sorely needed.

In general, cells interact with their surroundings using *receptors* at their surface – small protein molecules that protrude out from the cell – which bind other molecules either in the surrounding solution or on other cells. For T cells, there were two schools of thought. One was that T cells have a *single* receptor that could somehow recognize virus protein and MHC proteins together. The other was that these immune cells must have *two* receptors: one to recognize a virus protein and one to recognize the MHC protein. Both would have to be triggered to cause an immune response.

Different research groups raced to find out the nature of the receptor on T cells. Several made progress,[38] but the discovery that made things clear was the identification of the genes that encode the T-cell receptor. Mark Davis at the NIH and then Stanford did this using a technically difficult method which finds genes that T cells use and another cell type, say B cells, that don't.[39] Instrumental to his success was that he was thinking differently from everyone else – and he did a different kind of experiment from everyone else.

He wasn't thinking about how HLA proteins worked – or about the immune system per se – but was thinking instead about what makes a T cell different from another type of cell.[40] All the cells in one person's body contain the same set of genes, but different genes are 'switched on' to make proteins in different cells, giving each cell its unique appearance and role in the body. What Davis particularly wanted to know was which genes were specifically switched on in T cells. That way of thinking led him to find a gene that was variable between different T cells and never found in other cells – so it had to be the main receptor on T cells involved in the recognition of viruses.

He announced his discovery of the T-cell receptor genes in August 1983, in an impromptu talk at the World Immunology Congress in Kyoto, Japan. The journal *Science* took the highly unusual step of publishing a note on the meeting announcement in September 1983.[41] Normally, any scientific result has to be assessed by the scientists – the famous peer-review process – and this usually takes months. Indeed, Davis's discovery was properly published – after peer review – in March 1984.[42] The debate over the nature of the T-cell receptor was settled: there was one receptor that varied from one T cell to the next (allowing each T cell to detect one type of non-self molecule, such as one found on a germ).

But this only led to a new problem: how was this single T-cell receptor able to recognize the presence of a virus in conjunction with MHC protein? The very thing that Zinkernagel and Doherty discovered – that T cells would only detect a virus when it infected a cell with a particular MHC protein – was still mysterious. How this really works – at the level of what the T-cell receptor really detects on another cell – remained crucial to work out, both to fundamentally understand how the immune system worked and also for the aim to medically aid or hinder immune responses.

Again, opinions differed about how the T-cell receptor might work. One view was that the T-cell receptor recognized viral protein stuck or sitting next to HLA proteins. Another view was that a virus modified HLA protein in some way that could be recognized by the T-cell receptor. Nobody knew. And while uncovering the broad concepts of immunology gained much from mere thinking, the molecular details that make it work in practice were very hard to theorize about; simply, more experiments were needed. And another hero.

Alain Townsend was a twenty-three-year-old medic at St Mary's Hospital in London when he first read the 1974–5 papers by Zinkernagel and Doherty; he was blown away by their importance. Townsend was also fascinated by evidence that susceptibility to some diseases was known to correlate with the types of compatibility genes an individual inherited. So he began a PhD project at the National Institute for Medical Research in Mill Hill, London, to determine how T-cell recognition worked.[43] There was one fact that seemed especially puzzling to him – that some viruses could be detected by T cells even when the virus didn't have any of its own proteins at the cell surface. So how could they be detected?

Townsend and his colleague Andrew McMichael – both men calm, gentle and gifted in thinking clearly – had cultured T cells that could detect one particular 'flu protein. They had looked for this protein at the surface of 'flu-infected cells and were sure it wasn't there – it was only found inside cells. How could this protein be seen by T cells as a sign of disease on another cell if it isn't on the surface of the infected cell and is only found inside? Townsend and McMichael would often head to the local pub and thrash about ideas.[44]

Townsend carried out a pivotal set of experiments which spanned the early 1980s, as part of his PhD project in Mill Hill and continuing when he moved to Oxford University, working in a research institute linked to the John Radcliffe Hospital. In one pioneering experiment he compared how well T cells killed other cells that were treated in three different ways: firstly, cells were infected with the influenza virus; secondly, cells weren't infected with the whole virus but were engineered to make the one viral protein which the T cells responded to; thirdly, cells were engineered to only make bits of that one viral protein. This third variation was the most important part of the experiment; these cells did not contain influenza virus or even the one protein molecule which the T cells responded to – they just had bits of that protein, called peptides.

Townsend found that T cells could equally well kill cells treated in any of these three ways. He also established that different T cells were activated by different parts of the 'flu protein.[45] His follow-up to this is the experiment that is nowadays celebrated the most: instead of using cells engineered to make viral protein, or bits of viral protein, he just directly added to the cells bits of the viral protein – peptides – that had been synthetically made.[46] Over twenty-five years later, Townsend still vividly remembers the wondrous moment he looked down the microscope and saw that cells bathed in the right peptide had been destroyed by killer T cells.[47]

74

It was obvious that the cells had been killed: they simply came unstuck from the bottom of the dish. He showed McMichael, and they went to the pub to celebrate.[48] He knew the outcome of the experiment, but to get a result that was publishable – he couldn't just write that he *saw* cells being killed – he had to wait to get a precise answer from his experiment, measured as the amount of radioactivity released into the surrounding liquid as a result of radioactive cells being destroyed. Back from his drink, Townsend got these formal results. It confirmed what he had seen: his experiment apparently showed that killer T cells would recognize and destroy cells that had small viral peptides and a particular HLA protein. This was an astounding result: it showed that the immune system could tell that a cell was diseased if it contained just a small piece of one protein from a virus. That is, small fragments of protein, called peptides, are recognized as signs of disease by the immune system.

But not everyone agreed. Zinkernagel, for one, didn't like it, probably because there was no simple explanation as to how small parts of the viral protein would be recognized by T cells – this would only be solved when Bjorkman, Wiley and Strominger eventually presented a picture of what the HLA protein looks like, still eighteen months away. Scepticism from Zinkernagel hurt because young Townsend worshipped the ground he stood on.[49]

To resolve the matter, it was agreed that Townsend would send his cells to Zinkernagel's lab so that his team could repeat the experiments. Soon after, the pair met at a British Society of Immunology Congress, and Townsend tentatively inquired about the outcome. Zinkernagel said things didn't work out – he couldn't repeat the experiments that Townsend had published. Even worse, one of Zinkernagel's assistants had found out that all the cells sent by Townsend were contaminated with a type of bacteria called mycoplasma, which was known to make cells do strange things. It was a huge blow.

Townsend couldn't believe it. His laboratory was really careful not to get this type of contamination, and he felt so sure that he hadn't worked with contaminated cells. So he gently inquired who had done the experiments – and, came the answer, it was one of the junior medics in Zinkernagel's lab. OK, Townsend replied, I'll send the reagents and cells again – but this time you have to get somebody experienced in your lab to do it – or do it yourself.

It was a tense situation; there wasn't anything Townsend could do but wait. Talking to me in 2011, he recalls how he took solace in thinking about Galileo's 1610 publication, *The Starry Messenger*, how it caused a similar ruckus. Galileo had built a new 'spyglass' – or telescope, as it would later be called. With it, he saw many new stars and discovered four of Jupiter's moons. And he saw how the moon 'is not robed in a smooth and polished surface but is in fact rough and uneven, covered everywhere, just like the earth's surface, with huge prominences, deep valleys, and chasms'.[50] He even estimated that some lunar mountains were four miles tall. But, for everybody else, the moon looked smooth, and most just thought Galileo's observations bunkum. So Galileo made more spyglasses and sent them to some of the sceptics. Only then did it become accepted that the moon was not smooth.

For Townsend, the story had a twofold significance. It showed that the key to having a discovery accepted by others is both that the tools with which the discovery was made have to be shared and that the experiment has to be easy for others to do. If a result relies on extremely rare or new technology, it's very hard for others to validate it. Townsend's method to detect cells being destroyed (the so-called radioactive-release assay) was the same type of experiment that Zinkernagel had used in his Nobel-Prize-winning work with Doherty and was easy for any lab to perform.

The second round of experiments was a triumphant vindication of Townsend's discovery: from then on, Zinkernagel was a staunch supporter of his work. The combination of non-self-peptide with an HLA protein was essentially the 'altered self' that Zinkernagel and Doherty had discussed a decade earlier – the idea that a modification to the HLA protein is detected as a signature of disease. When Doherty first read Townsend's papers, he couldn't believe he'd missed the discovery for himself, and he thinks that, 'if they had named a third person on our Nobel, it should have been Alain [Townsend]'.[51]

But the mystery still remained in picturing clearly how HLA protein and a fragment of virus protein could activate T cells. How did this work? Bjorkman, Strominger and Wiley were on the verge of solving the problem – they had the raw data in hand – but the analysis to reveal the shape of the HLA protein was still difficult. Another postdoctoral researcher had joined Wiley's group, Mark Saper, and he did a lot of work in analysing Bjorkman's data.[52] Ninety per cent of the protein chain could be traced but there was that fuzzy 10 per cent yet to give up its secret. They didn't think that it could be a peptide like those that Townsend used, because Bjorkman made her crystals from pure HLA protein taken from cells that weren't infected with a virus.[53]

The moment of truth finally came in spring 1987. With all of HLA-A*02 accounted for, the troublesome fuzzy 10 per cent occupied a groove at the top of the HLA protein. It was positioned on top of a flat sheet of protein, cupped between two long helixes of HLA protein. The fuzziness was indeed the size of a peptide. The HLA protein, it transpired, was perfectly formed for clasping and displaying peptides.[54]

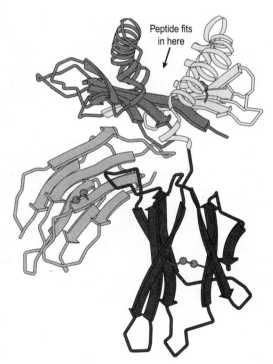

The shape of the HLA protein

As in most scientific breakthroughs, there wasn't a true eureka moment because calculating the protein structure was such a long process (at that time – it isn't any more). The structure is a beautiful one – appropriately enough, for it gets to the heart of how self and non-self discrimination really works.[55] Bjorkman had not added any viral or non-self peptide to her samples, yet in the groove at the top of the HLA protein sat a peptide. These peptides, Bjorkman reasoned, must have come from the cell itself – meaning that HLA protein associates with all kinds of peptides from inside the cell, not just non-self peptides.

This was an extraordinarily significant discovery. Until this point, most scientists had focused on understanding how HLA proteins combined with non-self peptides, from viruses and the like. But the structure showed that HLA doesn't discriminate between non-self and self peptides, it just binds all kinds of peptides, ones made by cells normally as well as others coming from a viral infection. There were hints of how HLA behaved in other studies going back many years – but precisely how it did so had remained hazy. Now, the picture of the HLA protein brought the way it worked into sharp focus.

What it revealed was this. All the protein molecules made inside your cells are continually being chopped up into peptides; these, in turn, are put up for show in the groove of HLA protein. In this way, a cell constantly 'reports' on its surface samples of all the proteins that it is making. T cells, meanwhile, have receptors that survey the pieces of protein that are put up for show, looking for anything 'non-self'. T cells then get activated when something appears that has never been in your body before. Recall that T cells are made so that each one has a unique receptor. They use these receptors to detect what is being held in the groove of the HLA proteins on another cell. Any self-reactive T cell – one that has a receptor that will be activated by a self-peptide in the groove of HLA protein – is killed off in the thymus, the organ once thought to be useless because it is just full of dead immune cells. So, any T cell let out of the thymus has a receptor that can be activated by a particular combination of peptide and HLA protein. If one of these T cells gets activated, it must have seen a peptide that has never been in your body before. This, in short, is how self and non-self are distinguished.

So significant was this discovery that Wiley ordered a communication lockdown. Nobody was to hear about it before their picture of the HLA protein was published. That meant that for two months there would be no talking about it at all: no conference papers or even informal chit-chat with other scientists about the data. Wiley's lockdown gave Bjorkman the difficulty of having to do job interviews in which she couldn't say what they had discovered. In these two months, Wiley and his colleagues produced two papers, one on the structure of the HLA protein itself[56] and another on the broad ramifications of the protein's shape.[57] Unsurprisingly, when they were submitted, both papers were accepted for publication in *Nature* within days, skipping the normal two to three months of back-and-forth peer review.

Strangely, prizes that followed celebrated different combinations of people from the trio involved.[58] But, in fact, each member of this trinity was essential for the breakthrough to have happened: Strominger had already worked for over fifteen years on HLA and it was crucial that his lab knew how to isolate and purify the HLA protein; Wiley had the necessary expertise in the X-ray technique used to actually get the structure; and it was the hard work and dedication of their PhD student Bjorkman that made it work over an eight-year-long scientific marathon. Even so, the trio didn't click together in the same way that Medawar's holy trinity did. Medawar was the undisputed leader of Billingham and Brent; here, instead, Wiley and Strominger were both ambitious leaders who came together to solve a problem while running independent research labs.

While Wiley and Strominger had half an eye on prizes, the main thing on Bjorkman's mind, beyond the science itself, was getting a job: the achievement won her a prestigious faculty position at Caltech in Pasadena, California, which she took up early in 1989. There she continues today, working on other structural studies with a view to medical applications. Aged in his late eighties, Strominger still runs a well-funded research programme at Harvard and is co-author on close to a thousand scientific papers. Zinkernagel has retired and mainly enjoys walking in the mountains, while Doherty continues in research and writes widely, recently publishing a book about global warming.[59]

A month after Wiley's disappearance, a crane operator saw his body bob up between some logs in the Mississippi River, 340 miles downstream from Memphis. The subsequent inquest considered murder – by terrorists – and suicide, but eventually determined on a verdict of accidental death. The sequence of events was held to have gone as follows. Wiley had been drinking at the hospital banquet and left late to drive to his father's house nearby, instead of staying overnight in the hotel along with the other guests. There was long delay between his leaving the banquet and his car arriving at the bridge. Somewhere along the way, he probably took a wrong turning. He had slightly dented the car, maybe as he tried to turn it around on the bridge. Maybe he got out of the car to check the damage or maybe he got out to vomit. Whatever the reason, the police concluded that he was then blown off the bridge, probably by a truck whizzing by or a sudden gust of wind. Wiley was tall and the bridge had a low bar that would have come up only to his thigh. A key piece of evidence was a button found on a beam of the bridge. If he had jumped, he would easily have cleared the beam.

Who knows what knowledge we lost when Wiley died, like the unsung melodies gone when John Lennon was shot? From January 1996 to October 1999 I worked with Strominger at Harvard, in the same building as Wiley. I occasionally ran into Wiley and now back in the UK I often wonder if he realized how far his research, his teaching and his persona stretched out in front of him, affecting people like me, who knew him only slightly. Do any of us ever realize that? We connect in myriad ways; from the impact of what each of us say and do every day to the common thread of our genetic inheritance that we are only beginning to understand.

PART TWO

The Frontier of Compatibility Gene Research

5

Differences between Us That Matter

How important are our differences in compatibility genes? The brief answer is that these genes influence if and how fast you recover from almost any disease you may get. This chapter will explain this fully, but first, to gain perspective, it helps to consider the impact of our genetic inheritance on our well-being in general.

There's no clearer example of how dramatic an effect genes *can* have on one's health and behaviour than in the life of Woody Guthrie, the American folk singer, left-wing observer of the Great Depression, and inspiration to Bob Dylan and Bruce Springsteen. Guthrie played a guitar scrawled with the words 'This machine kills fascists', reputedly wrote over a thousand songs and published an intoxicating autobiography, *Bound for Glory*, an ode to living free, riding freight trains and personal rebelliousness.[1] But Guthrie suffered gravely from a genetic mutation; his daughter Nora never knew him as healthy.[2] While he was in his thirties, when he should have been at the peak of success, his behaviour became erratic and even violent.

On the evening of 15 May 1952 he attacked his wife, Nora's mother, Marjorie. She had come into the house to find him strangely glazed over and holding scissors. He'd cut the telephone wire; the attack was premeditated. Marjorie got upstairs, onto the bed, but he followed and began pummelling her with his fists. Something was very strange, and he seemed to be frothing at the mouth. This attack was crazier than ever before, and Marjorie distinctly noticed that he was sober. She escaped to get the neighbours' attention, and the police arrived not a moment too soon. When an officer said he knew Guthrie's songs, things quietened. Marjorie, having just experienced hell, told the truth: 'Woody, you're sick . . . I don't know what it is and you don't know what it is, but you're sick.'[3]

The next day Guthrie checked into hospital on a three-week programme for alcoholics and, once out of hospital, he wrote to Marjorie to try to convince her that it was just liquor that turned him into a senseless raving idiot.[4] Finally, on 3 September 1952, a neurologist realized that Guthrie had Huntington's disease. Until that point, his tics, shakes and slurred speech had just been taken as eccentric mannerisms of a great artist. Lost in illness, one day in May 1956 he was arrested for not having a bus ticket, and police took him to Greystone Psychiatric Hospital, New Jersey, where he would stay for many years. Bob Dylan visited him there to bring cigarettes and play songs – first in January 1961[5] – and remembers how 'it was a strange environment to meet anybody, least of all the true voice of the American spirit . . . The experience was sobering and psychologically draining.'[6]

After Guthrie's death – on 3 October 1967, when he was fifty-five – Marjorie took out an ad in the *New York Times* to bring afflicted families together. She persuaded US President Jimmy Carter to set up a commission for studying neurological diseases. This led to the founding of the Huntington's Disease Society of America, which raised money for the research that led to the first genetic markers of the disease. Marjorie died in 1983 but the Woody Guthrie Folk Festival, held in Oklahoma each July, raises money for more research. It includes an annual pancake breakfast run by Woody's younger sister Mary Jo, who by chance didn't inherit her brother's illness.[7] Eventually, in 1993, the single gene that underlies Huntington's disease was discovered.[8]

The normal version of this gene has a section in which a small stretch is repetitive. In the disease-causing mutant, this repeated part of the gene is longer than normal, so cells then produce a version of the protein that's bigger than normal, and this leads to cognitive problems and dementia – although exactly why this is remains unclear. Speech and many higher brain functions commonly deteriorate, although long-term memory is spared, not necessarily making life any happier. As many as one in four patients attempt suicide; depression is common.[9]

Because a single copy of the mutant gene is enough to cause the disease, then, if one parent has it, their child simply has a 50 per cent chance of inheriting it. Children often witness one of their parents suffering, knowing there's a chance their fate is similar. Some choose to know for certain by taking a genetic test; some don't. The question – to know or not to know – eats away at many for much of their lives. You can only gain certain knowledge whether you will inevitably get the disease or not; there's no cure.

Cystic fibrosis is another well-known genetic disease, one of the most common potentially lethal genetic disorders for European Caucasians. The difference from Huntington's is that for cystic fibrosis people can carry one dysfunctional copy of the gene without any symptoms because they still have another, normal, version that compensates. Disease arises only when a person inherits two copies of the impaired gene. That means that, if each parent has a copy of the mutant gene, there's a one in four chance their child will inherit cystic fibrosis. Inheriting two aberrant copies of the cystic fibrosis gene leaves people unable to correctly make a particular protein which normally helps salt move in and out of cells. Loss or inefficiency of this protein has an effect on many organs which leads to a range of symptoms such as difficulty breathing following a lung infection. Shortly before he became the UK's prime minister in 2007, Gordon Brown's new-born son Fraser was diagnosed with cystic fibrosis. Brown rarely discusses it in public, but in one interview he said what anyone would think at some point in the face of such difficulty: 'We sometimes say: well, why, why, why, why us? You know, why did this happen to us?'[10] Science can't give an answer as to why any one particular person is affected – but one of the great triumphs of human biology is that we do have an explanation as to why some disease-causing mutations are kept in the population at all.

Sickle cell anaemia is a powerful example where this is clear. This disease comes from inheriting a mutant version of haemoglobin – a protein in red blood cells that binds oxygen to release it where appropriate around the body. A change in one of the haemoglobin genes gives rise to an altered protein, haemoglobin S. The presence of haemoglobin S changes red blood cells from their normal disc-like shape into an abnormally curved 'sickle' shape, which makes them fragile and interferes with their circulation through small blood vessels. Those who inherit one copy of haemoglobin S produce both normal and abnormal haemoglobin. This doesn't cause a life-threatening problem, as there is still enough normal haemoglobin to transport oxygen around the body. People with one copy of this gene simply have to take care when oxygen might be in short supply, at high altitude for example. However, an inheritance of two copies leads to sickle cell anaemia, which can cause damage to several organs and early death. Despite this danger, the mutation turns out to be surprisingly common in sub-Saharan Africa. For example, in Nigeria about one in four people carry a copy of the haemoglobin S gene. There are tribal variations – 45 per cent of people in the Baamba tribe in the west of Uganda, for example, carry it.[11] Why is this potentially lethal mutation found in *so* many people?

The first clue to answering this came from mapping where people have haemoglobin S; the area where people have this gene has a striking resemblance to the distribution of malaria. This fits with haemoglobin S providing protection against malaria. Even within the same geographical region of Africa, haemoglobin S is common in people living in lowlands but relatively rare in people indigenous to the highlands, where malaria is not endemic, because mosquitoes don't live that high up. In fact, we now know that the sickle cell trait caused by haemoglobin S can be 90 per cent protective against severe and complicated forms of malaria, and that's why the mutant gene is retained in the population.

So this specific genetic mutation protects us against one major disease, malaria, at a cost of some people inheriting two copies and getting sickle cell anaemia. That is, there's one reason to keep the gene – it helps against malaria – and one reason to get rid of it – as it makes people susceptible to anaemia. So it's kept in the population at a frequency dependent on balancing the level of threat from these two diseases. Where malaria is endemic, such as in West African lowlands, the mutation is retained, because having it makes you more likely to have and raise healthy children. In populations living without malaria, such as in the African highlands, the mutation is very rare. In short, the outcome is human diversity.

So just how diverse are all the genes we each have? Roughly speaking, humans are 99.9 per cent the same genetically – just 0.1 per cent of genes varies from person to person. You might guess that the *most* variable genes among us would be those that influence hair type, eye colour, or skin pigmentation. But, in fact, the genes that vary most between people don't affect anything superficially obvious at all. Those that vary the most are our immune-system genes – especially our compatibility genes. Why are these genes so enormously diverse – and why does it matter which ones you have?

The early pioneers of human compatibility genes – Dausset, van Rood, Payne and the others we met in Chapter 3 – wondered whether or not our variation in these genes linked with disease. They were encouraged by studies in animals, where data was easier to interpret because of inbred strains of mice – one influential study, for example, reported in 1964 that different strains of mice varied in their susceptibility to a type of leukaemia caused by a virus.[12] In humans, the first link between HLA and disease was established for a type of white blood cell cancer, Hodgkin's lymphoma, in 1972. But it is only a small effect; people with Hodgkin's lymphoma have a slightly increased chance of having certain HLA genes.[13]

Unlike the genes that underlie Huntington's, cystic fibrosis or sickle cell anaemia, HLA is not an all-or-nothing mark of disease. Single genes that underlie disease are very rare; most illnesses are complex and involve both genetic and environmental factors. Virtually all cancers, for example, have been linked to specific genetic variants but having certain mutations doesn't usually make cancer inevitable. Your chance of getting the associated cancer can be increased by a particular genetic inheritance, but usually cancer still remains a small risk overall. Likewise, the compatibility genes you have inherited make you more susceptible to some diseases and more resistant to others – but usually to a small extent.

This in itself causes a problem in testing for connections between HLA and disease. Because HLA is so diverse – and its effects are subtle – one version of an HLA gene can easily show up just by chance as being unusually frequent in a particular set of people with a specific disease. That is, any single study can quite easily give a false indication that one HLA type is associated with a particular disease or trait.[14] This needs to be taken into account by using a statistical analysis more complex than used in everyday lab experiments. Another problem is that any small effects detected could be due to unknown genes nearby or connected to HLA genes, rather than HLA itself.

That's why, historically, consensus about which HLA types genuinely associate with a disease has been hard to reach. The early pioneers struggled to convince everyone about the importance of HLA in disease. Eventually, in 1973, a clear link between HLA and disease was established by two groups – one in the US and one in the UK – who reported their discoveries almost at the same time. Although other links between HLA and disease had been indicated, this one was dramatic.

In the US, Rodney Bluestone, Paul Terasaki and their colleagues in the University of California Los Angeles (UCLA) discovered that 88 per cent of people with ankylosing spondylitis had HLA-B*27, whereas its frequency in the general population was just 8 per cent.[15] Ankylosing spondylitis is an autoimmune disease that leads to inflammation within joints, especially in the spine. It had been studied for over a century but little progress had been made in deciphering its causes. Strangely, the UCLA team's breakthrough finding was rejected for publication by the top medical journal the *Lancet*.[16] Instead, they published their work in the *New England Journal of Medicine*, only to then see that another group, led by Derrick Brewerton at Westminster Hospital, London, had the same conclusion published in the *Lancet* – the very same journal which had just rejected their paper.[17] Why the *Lancet* rejected one study and published another with the same conclusion is unfortunately not known. Terasaki has suggested that anyway he was first in the discovery, evidenced by his team's abstract from a conference in November 1972 being the first publication of the finding.[18] In contrast, Brewerton regards the outcome of this race as a dead heat.[19] For science, the real value of having the result confirmed in two independent studies was that it immediately gave everyone confidence in the conclusion; together, these two studies unequivocally established for everyone that HLA does influence disease.

The UCLA team had been fully engaged in HLA research for over a decade – Terasaki was one of the HLA pioneers involved in the early international meetings, and he developed a widely used method for testing HLA types. Brewerton's paper, on the other hand, seemed to come out of the blue; he was a clinical rheumatologist, entirely unknown to HLA scientists. His only previous contribution to immunology was indirect: he had helped treat Peter Medawar after his stroke and was the target of Medawar's anger when told that he should learn to write with his left hand as his right side may not recover.[20]

Brewerton's contribution to the story of our compatibility genes began one summer's day in 1971, when he happened to sit down for lunch opposite the head of his hospital's tissue-typing facility, who had just returned from a conference where there was a lot of discussion about the possibility that HLA could associate with disease. From that discussion Brewerton realized that he should test the HLA types of patients with ankylosing spondylitis, because it was known that an inherited factor was important in this disease, and nobody knew what it was. A grant application on the idea was rejected, but some hospital funds became available to employ someone to help in tissue-typing, which gave them the opportunity for research around their clinical duties. 'As a result,' Brewerton remembers, 'I often started work in my office at 4am and stopped only when the library closed at night. Family life went on hold.'[21]

Why was this so pioneering? Because it was a time when thinking about genes didn't permeate our culture as deeply as it does now. So, although it was clear that certain diseases congregated in families, many clinicians didn't think it a top priority to find out which genes associate with arthritic diseases. Brewerton tested eight patients and found that all of them had HLA-B*27, a probability of happening by chance of less than one in a million. He felt that he was on to the most important discovery ever made in understanding arthritis.[22]

Brewerton decided that he next needed to plan a military-style operation to test a hundred patients and several control groups. It was before computers were widely used, so there weren't databases of patients to call upon. He recruited patients by asking, across thirty-seven hospitals, if doctors could recall anyone appropriate for his study – 'all done in a very primitive way', he later recalled.[23] The results were astonishing – 24 out of 25 patients had HLA-B*27, then 48 out of 50. Brewerton was elated, but he was also very afraid; it just seemed too good to be true.[24]

Losing sleep at night, he kept thinking of problems: what if something unknown, a new virus perhaps, caused the disease, and this new thing somehow interfered with the HLA test to give a false reading of B*27 being present? Or what if some of the drugs used for treatment somehow influenced the HLA tests to give false readings? In hindsight, these worries seem overly cautious; theoretically feasible but beyond reasonable doubt. Yet the anxiety is almost inevitable for any conscientious scientist going over every possible alternative interpretation of their data before being sure their discovery is right. Eventually, Brewerton found a way out.

He decided to test the HLA type of each patient's close relatives – because some of these relatives should also have inherited B*27 even when they don't have the disease. That way he would know his tests were giving the correct HLA type, and not a result of something strange in people with ankylosing spondylitis. Brewerton travelled all over London, visiting families to collect blood samples, usually very early each morning.[25] It took a few unnerving months, but he finally confirmed that family members also had B*27, even when they did not show signs of illness. Brewerton's fog of fear cleared, and he accepted that his team had proven that someone who had inherited HLA-B*27 was about 300 times more likely to develop ankylosing spondylitis. After publishing, Brewerton learned of the UCLA results, and his reaction was disappointment that he had not made the discovery alone.[26]

The US team – Bluestone and Terasaki – had arrived at the same discovery by a very different route. Born to a poor immigrant family in Los Angeles in 1929, Terasaki spent most of his career at UCLA, where, in 1964, he established a test for HLA types that could use very small samples of blood. Over the following few years, he and his team automated this method so that hundreds of HLA tests could be done in a day. This enabled him to set up an ambitious programme to study huge numbers of patients, searching for unusual frequencies of HLA types in all kinds of diseases. One of the diseases he tested, with clinician Rodney Bluestone, was gout.

For something to compare with gout, they decided to use patients with another rheumatic disease, ankylosing spondylitis. It was these control patients that turned out to be more interesting than they planned – not a blank control at all – and the link between B*27 and ankylosing spondylitis was revealed. Serendipity played a big role for both teams: Terasaki's team chose interesting patients as a comparison to the disease they actually set out to study, and Brewerton had sat down to lunch in just the right place.

From here, Terasaki's and Brewerton's careers couldn't have diverged any further. Brewerton remained focused on clinical duties, wrote a book about arthritis,[27] and later chaired a local campaign group set up to protect a small beach near his Sussex home.[28] Terasaki, on the other hand, founded, in 1984, a company called One Lambda to sell the tools needed for tissue-typing; as a result, in 2010, he could donate $50 million to UCLA. When I met Brewerton at age eighty-seven, in 2011, he said that he no longer thinks about his work on HLA-B*27, that it all seems very distant – like it happened to someone else.[29]

The fact that so many people with this disease have B*27 is striking, but it's also important to realize that if you have B*27 you are still very unlikely to get the disease. Other genes and environmental factors are also important, so that, overall, it's not very useful to have a genetic test for B*27, because it's not strongly predictive of disease on its own. It can perhaps have a role in diagnosing ankylosing spondylitis if symptoms are mild or ambiguous, but the main impact of the B*27 discovery has been scientific; a stepping stone to understanding our HLA system.

Later, it was discovered that people with HLA-B*27 are also more susceptible to the skin disease psoriasis and an inflammation of the eye known as uveitis. This meant that the same compatibility gene could make someone susceptible to a range of diseases that are clinically very different. Then, around thirty-five years after the ankylosing spondylitis story broke, B*27 hit the limelight again. A monumental project involving over 200 different research centres found that B*27 was linked to Acquired Immunodeficiency Syndrome (AIDS) – but this time it *protected* against the illness.

People infected with HIV don't progress to AIDS at the same rate. The general course of events following infection is that the virus multiplies dramatically in the first few weeks and 'flu-like symptoms develop. By about four weeks, the immune system starts to lower the amount of virus in the blood, until it reaches a steady level about two months later. The number of copies of the virus in a person's blood then stays level over a period called the chronic phase of infection, and during this time patients don't seem ill at all, although they can still infect others. Later, virus numbers increase and AIDS develops – but how long this takes varies considerably. Some succumb quickly, whereas others infected with the virus can stay free of the disease for many years.

A fortunate few – about 1 in 10 – stay disease-free for a very long time – more than seven years. They are known as the Long Term Non-Progressors. But about 1 in 300 is even luckier than that. Their immune system can attack the virus to such an extent that it becomes almost entirely undetectable. They are the HIV Controllers or the Elite Controllers. In the battle against AIDS, these few individuals have superpowers endowed by their genes.

HLA genes were first linked with resistance to AIDS in 1996 – although this first study involved a relatively small number of patients.[30] HLA-B*57 was found to occur far more frequently in patients that do not rapidly progress to AIDS.[31] But one criticism of this research in the 1990s – as with all research into HLA and disease at that time – was that these data didn't establish how important the link to HLA was *in comparison to other genes*. Nowadays, all of the genes can be compared across many individuals with or without a particular trait or disease. This approach – called a genome-wide association study, or GWAS – has found genetic variations that affect a range of human traits, including our height, body mass index and blood lipid levels. A first GWAS for HIV *indicated* that regions of the genome at or near HLA were associated with lower levels of virus in a patient's blood.[32] Then the International HIV Controllers Study – a study led by Bruce Walker at Massachusetts General Hospital and Paul de Bakker at Harvard University – aimed to pin down exactly which genes were important.

Walker had been building up to this moment for twenty-five years, having first submitted an application to study our immune response to HIV in 1985. At that time, his application was rejected because – as the committee told him – HIV *suppresses* our immune response, so what could be the point in studying our immune response to it? But, after being inspired by reading Alain Townsend's research – the work we discussed in Chapter 4, that HLA proteins present bits of proteins or peptides from viruses – Walker applied for funding again. His application was rejected a second time, along with the clarification: Dr Walker, you really don't get it – this is an immune suppressive illness and we told you before.[33]

Two decades later, however, one couple's donation of $100 million freed Walker to pursue his dreams.[34] He had recently accompanied philanthropist Terry Ragon to Africa to visit AIDS patients with a view to raising money for HIV research, the kind of trip he'd done several times before. In 1978, Ragon had founded a company to provide database software which became the source of his fortune. After their trip to Africa together, Walker mentioned that he thought progress was hampered by research being fragmented in silos: that teams studying different aspects of HIV didn't mix. Ragon reckoned out loud that an institute to bring everyone together might require $10 million a year over ten years, and then casually added: and my wife and I would like to give that to you.[35] The remark triggered an out-of-body experience for Walker.

He knew that this kind of flexible money would be entirely transformative. But his elation was quickly followed by sheer terror – with such a huge amount of money comes great responsibility.[36] In fact, Walker proved adept at raising money and he obtained several charitable donations – in effect establishing his own funding agency. One of the first studies to come from the Ragon Institute, with its many collaborating centres, was the HIV Controllers Study.[37]

In this huge study, 3,622 HIV-infected people of different ethnicities were divided up according to whether or not they were HIV Controllers – that is, according to whether or not they had maintained very low levels of virus in their blood after being infected, on average, ten years earlier. Their genomes were scanned, and the only statistically strong characteristic of HIV Controllers was in their compatibility genes. Carefully analysing that region of the genome revealed precise details; that having HLA-B*57, -27 or -14 is protective against AIDS, whereas having HLA-B*35 or HLA-Cw*07 associates with fast progression to AIDS.[38]

There were earlier studies showing that HLA genes influence the progression to AIDS,[39] including the identification of B*57 as being important,[40] but the scale of this study was new. By looking across the whole human genome, this study clarified that our HLA genes have the biggest influence in the human genome. Indeed, *only* the variations in our compatibility genes were significant when the whole genome was assessed.[41] This establishes that the very same genes that control the success of, say, a kidney transplant, influence how long we live after infection with HIV – two aspects of human biology that, at a glance, seem entirely unrelated.

While it might be a stretch to consider these genes as endowing superpowers, on the other hand, what is a superpower if it's not a rare ability to survive something that destroys others unfailingly? Genetic variation can't endow anyone an ability to fly like in the X-men comic books, but a real-life genetic superpower is that some of us can survive a deadly virus. How is this possible?

The answer lies in the details of how our HLA proteins work. Recall Townsend's experiments, the ones initially doubted by Zinkernagel. They showed that HLA proteins present samples of what's being made inside our cells – peptides – that can be scrutinized by our immune cells – T cells. The picture of the HLA protein – hard-won by Bjorkman, Strominger and Wiley – showed that peptides were clasped in a groove at the top of the HLA protein. In fact, there are about 100,000 of these HLA proteins on a cell's surface, so collectively they present a good sampling of what's currently being made inside. And detection of diseased cells occurs because a T cell can react to a peptide present in the groove of an HLA protein that hasn't been in your body before.

Bjorkman's pictures of HLA-A*02 – and the pictures of other HLA proteins that other teams obtained later – revealed another killer fact. Our differences in compatibility genes encode for slight variations in the HLA proteins we have – and pictures of HLA proteins showed that our differences are not positioned randomly throughout the protein's shape.[42] The bits of, say, HLA-A*02 and HLA-B*27 that are different are at the top of the molecule – in and around the groove where the peptides sit. This is a revelatory finding: it means that *each type of HLA gene makes a protein with a slightly different-shaped groove on top.*

Why is this so critical? Because this means that each type of HLA protein is best at clasping certain peptides – not all the ones that a cell might have. Put another way, each type of HLA protein presents a different sampling of what's being made inside a cell. And, most important of all, this means that for any particular peptide – say one that's produced in large amounts by a specific virus – only some HLA types of all those present in the population will be good at clasping it. So each person is better or worse at detecting any one particular peptide – according to which type of HLA proteins they have inherited.

HLA proteins that can't hold on to one particular peptide will have the right-shaped groove for others – perhaps one from another virus or an alternative peptide made by the same virus. Any one particular virus will encode many peptides, each of which can be used by many types of HLA proteins, but another factor to consider here is that certain combinations of peptides and HLA protein are particularly good at triggering a T-cell response. For example, a particular peptide may bind especially well to one type of HLA protein, which in turn strongly activates the appropriate T cells. The upshot of all this is that some of us will be inherently better than others at defending against a particular infection, such as one type of virus.

Back to our battle with HIV: this virus is especially hard for the immune system to attack, mainly because there's actually an enormous variation in the virus itself. The number of different versions of HIV in one infected person is greater than the variety in influenza virus seen worldwide in any one season.[43] When one version of HIV causes an infection, it takes only a few days for there to be immense variety – because, as the virus multiplies, it makes copies that are each slightly different. Variation in the virus helps it escape any particular attack from human T cells.

Each T cell, as we've seen, detects the virus by recognizing a particular peptide that it makes. So that means that each T cell will attack all forms of the virus that make a particular peptide – but other versions of the virus survive. As one HIV peptide provokes an attack by T cells, the pool of virus in that patient will be replaced by versions of the virus that don't make that particular peptide. In other words, the virus evolves inside us – changing its parts – to avoid attacks by our immune system. And that's why it's really hard for us to get rid of it.

In that case, why are some types of HLA proteins better than others in fighting HIV? Our HLA proteins grasp different peptides – chopped-up pieces of protein made by the HIV virus – but, crucially, some of these peptides are better than others for our immune system to detect. There are two reasons for this. The first is that it helps if the peptide comes from a protein that the virus makes a lot of. That way, there's an abundance of it available for T cells to see, triggering a strong reaction. The second reason is subtle – but actually more important.

Although the virus can change and produce many different versions, some parts of the virus are just so critical that they can't be altered: changing these parts would render the virus unable to work properly. This means that there are some bits of the virus that are the same across all the variants of HIV. So the second thing about a peptide that makes it a really good target for our immune system is if it is made from one of these *conserved* parts of the virus. If the immune system can detect one of these peptides, there aren't versions of the virus that can escape detection.

So the HLA types that are best at fighting a virus are those that can hold peptides made in large amounts from conserved parts of the virus. It turns out that HLA-B* 57 is good at binding a particular peptide from a conserved part of an abundant HIV protein (called Gag). And so it makes sense that HLA-B* 57 is found in around 30–50 per cent of HIV Controllers, five to ten times more frequently than it's found generally.

A warning: this is research in progress. And presentation of particular peptides by B* 57, for example, may not be the *sole* way in which HIV Controllers avoid AIDS but it is (almost certainly) a major factor. B* 27 is also one of the HLA types frequent in HIV Controllers, and yet this same genetic variation is part of the problem in ankylosing spondylitis – discovered by Brewerton and Terasaki. That is, the very same HLA that is good for us in dealing with one disease, HIV, is bad for us by contributing to another disease, ankylosing spondylitis. The role that B* 27 has in the auto-immune disease ankylosing spondylitis is (almost certainly) also a result of its job of presenting peptides to T cells. But in this case, normal self-peptides – chopped-up pieces of protein found in healthy cells – are wrongly identified as non-self and trigger an immune response. This gives rise to the auto-immune disease – because our immune system makes a mistake and attacks healthy tissue.

But why would one particular type of HLA gene underlie this kind ~~of autoimm.~~
of disease? The short answer is that nobody really knows. It could be
that B*27 binds an abundant self-peptide extremely well and this
leads to problems. Or alternatively, there could be some real non-self
peptide, say from a virus, presented by B*27 to activate T cells, which
then accidentally attack uninfected cells by responding to a self-peptide
that just happens to be similar to the one from the virus.[44] Even
though we don't understand exactly how B*27 is involved in ankylosing spondylitis, there's plenty of evidence that, in general, T cells and
HLA genes are important in many auto-immune diseases. Class II ~~Type I~~
compatibility genes designated HLA-DR*03 and -DR*04 are found ~~Diabetes~~
in the vast majority of people with type I diabetes, for example. In
fact, virtually the whole gamut of possible illnesses that could ever
affect us are known to be influenced by our compatibility genes –
including cancer, infections, auto-immune diseases and even some
neurological disorders. HLA-B*53 can protect against severe malaria, for example, by binding a particular peptide made by the
parasite.[45] And other compatibility genes are linked to multiple sclerosis, Parkinson's, Hodgkin's lymphoma, inflammatory bowel disease,
leprosy, narcolepsy and so on.

By controlling our response to disease, our compatibility genes
influence how we live, when we die – and from what we die. Even so,
it's important to keep in mind that, even though many Elite Controllers of HIV have HLA-B*27, having this type of HLA is *not sufficient*
to survive AIDS. There is still much to be learned about our immune
response to HIV and other infections. And, whatever HLA type you
have inherited, by far the best way to stay safe is to avoid being
infected in the first place.

The compatibility gene system doesn't only explain how any one of
us might fare better or worse against a particular disease like AIDS.
It is a far bigger system than that. It also works between us all, across
the whole human species, because our immune system has evolved in
defence of humanity as a whole – to protect all of us as a species from
anything dangerous that could arise.

As we've seen, these genes vary from person to person, and across
the human population there are billions of combinations of HLA
types possible. In fact, it's theoretically possible for everyone on the

planet to have a different set of HLA genes. This doesn't quite happen because some HLA types are more common than others, but there is still enormous diversity in the population. This means that a virus escaping detection by the HLA proteins in one individual will face different HLA types in someone else. If we were all infected with one especially deadly virus, for example, some of us may survive by having a particularly potent HLA type for dealing with that virus. An outcome of this is that the distribution of HLA types among us evolves over time, as waves of different infections influence who reproduces.

But if some HLA genes are better at fighting a particular infection – because they can pick up appropriate peptides – then why do we each have only six class I HLA genes, for example? Why don't we each have hundreds or thousands of HLAs like the whole population does? If a virus has managed to avoid detection via one HLA type, it's useful to have another that may work. So hundreds or thousands of HLA genes in each person would surely be better at catching all possible infections, wouldn't they?

It's hard to do an experiment to answer this, but the generally accepted theory is that the system has a limit because of the way our body discriminates self and non-self. Recall that any T cell capable of reacting to ourselves is killed off in the thymus. That implies that, for each HLA type, all the T cells reacting to self peptides clasped by that type of HLA protein have to be killed off. Too many HLA types and it would be hard to have a big enough pool of T cells left. So there is a balance between maximizing the number of non-self peptides that can be grabbed by HLA, while still allowing enough T cells to exist for the detection of all possible non-self peptides. Or, in broader terms, there is delicate balance in making sure the immune system cannot attack our own bodies yet can respond to all kinds of potential infections. The outcome of this balancing act is that our HLA type makes each of us more susceptible or resistant to different diseases – not like the individual genetic mutations which cause cystic fibrosis or Huntington's; compatibility genes influence our response to *all kinds of diseases*.

From this depth of understanding, the next question is pragmatic: how do we get to new cures?

6

A Path to New Medicine

The urgent debate in universities and pharmaceutical companies alike is about how to get the best out of the knowledge we've accumulated, how to translate revelations in our understanding of genetics and disease into actual medical benefit. Many of our best medicines so far have been vaccinations, but development of a vaccine for HIV, for example, has proved to be a long and bumpy ride ever since the US health secretary suggested in 1984 that it would take a couple more years. The discovery of HIV Controllers is encouraging for vaccine development, because these people show us that immune responses at least have the potential to control HIV in the right circumstances. If we could get other HLA types to be as potent as, say, HLA-B*57, then more people might join those who inherited superpowers.

There's no shortage of scientists trying to translate our knowledge into practical outcomes; conferences about HIV nowadays gather about 20,000 professionals and 2,000 journalists. Such meetings are not unlike *Star Trek* conventions; the passion is the same and the heroes are equally revered. Both are ignited by imagination and wonder. But the paramount fact distinguishing scientists from their science-fiction counterparts is that they are also driven by an important real cause: to create new medicines.

Some – Nobel laureate Rolf Zinkernagel is one – think the key issue in getting to new medicines is to perform experiments in which everything is as close as possible to being physiologically right: using animals, real viruses and doses that would occur naturally.[1] Others – such as Ron Germain, a leading scientist at the NIH – agrees that this is important but also advocates other approaches, such as computer simulations of immune responses.[2] The difficulty is that it's relatively easy to do something new; very hard to do something important, because, as Einstein put it, 'Not everything that can be counted counts.' My view is that, since the very essence of discovery is that nobody predicted it, who's to know what's best to do next?

In truth, many of the drugs that we use today were found by chance – or at least serendipitously. The discovery of antibiotics is a well-known example: on 28 September 1928, Alexander Fleming noticed that a fungus had contaminated one of his experiments and killed off the bacteria he was studying. A more recent example is Viagra, developed as a drug for high blood pressure and then later discovered to be of use in preventing erectile dysfunction. It has proved difficult, and all too rare, to systematically translate our knowledge into direct medical benefit. Sport commentators call something 'academic' when it's not important, but this issue is anything but 'academic'; our well-being and even our survival depend on us choosing the right path to new ways of conquering disease. So are there radically different approaches we could take?

Eric Schadt is one leading scientist who says there is. Renowned for turning up to meetings in shorts whatever the weather or formality of the occasion, he argues that molecular biology has been great for uncovering individual genes important for human traits but that we've largely failed to fulfil the medical promises that have been touted – and it's enough already. He argues that the main problem is that we haven't adequately tackled the *complexity* of genes and disease.

In general, many genes – not one – contribute to a disease risk or human trait. As we've seen, compatibility genes influence our susceptibility and resistance to all manner of diseases, but they don't fully protect against, or absolutely cause, any one. There are exceptions such as Huntington's disease, which is caused by a single genetic variant, but by and large things are more complicated than one gene causing one disease or trait. Studies of how frequently twins share an illness are one way in which we can estimate the total effect that genes have. And in comparison to the sum of the individual genes known to be important, we can account for only about 10 per cent of the total genetic risk for many human traits and diseases.[3] So, Schadt says, something big is missing in our understanding of genes and disease.

Einstein

Genome-wide associations studies have worked well in identifying many important genes. But even these huge studies – scanning the genes of thousands of people – are not perfect. Things that aren't easily picked up include rare genetic variants and modifications to our DNA made after birth (so-called epigenetic changes) and differences we can sometimes have in the number of copies of a given gene. But most important of all is that genes interact – the status of one influences another, and so on – like computer, social and financial networks. And variation in groups of genes is hard to analyse – only the effect of individual genes is easily studied.

So, Schadt, and others like him, suggests that a seismic shift in our approach is needed because most diseases involve interactions between constellations of genes. And things are even more complex than you might think at first because the interactions between genes are affected by diet, age, gender, exposure to toxins and so on.[4] Schadt's close colleague Stephen Friend, a paediatric oncologist, says it plainly: 'Traditional human disease research models are now archaic. The academic [grant] process is choked by favourite gene efforts that result primarily in "impactful" journal articles . . . And the patients? They're getting more and more frustrated.'[5] Yesteryear's revolution in biology was the Human Genome Project; Schadt wants to deliver the next one.

There's always a personal story behind the approach a scientist takes. Schadt's almost anarchic attitude – and his ability to weather a storm – was undoubtedly shaped by a series of fights early in his life.[6] His Christian parents brought him up, with his six siblings, with the attitude that secular education was worthless. Going to college was frowned upon, and Schadt joined the air force. But an accident while rappelling down a rockface left him with poor mobility in his shoulder, and he was told his role in the military would have to change. Having done well in various aptitude tests, in 1986, aged nineteen, he went to college after all. Physical exertion had been Schadt's release, but once he was at college, ideas and academic challenges became a new source of freedom. His religious upbringing helped focus his mind on big issues – how things are connected, underlying principles – and he was drawn to studying maths and philosophical logic. But by pursuing a college education his father considered he had become possessed by the devil; he told his son that he should never return home.[7]

Estranged from his family, Schadt had to fight to stay away from the military – after realizing that he had, in fact, been overwhelmingly depressed there – because they were paying for his education and expected him to return. Eventually he got a PhD from UCLA in 1999, and by that time he had already begun working at the pharmaceutical giant Roche. It was a time when large-scale analysis of genes was fairly new, and Roche was using a specific process for analysing genetic data which used machines purchased from another company, Affymetrix. Schadt wasn't happy that Affymetrix wouldn't let anyone see the computer codes being used to analyse the genetic data. It meant that he couldn't fiddle with it to tailor it to his specific needs. So he wrote his own software, which won him fame within Roche. But he grew tired of corporate meetings and decided to move to a small start-up company based in Seattle. Then, in November 1999 – a week before Schadt left Roche – things got ugly.

The first trace of trouble came when Schadt tried to remotely access his office computer but couldn't. He called his wife and asked if she could go to his office and check it. Maybe it had been turned off by mistake? She went in and found everything in his office had disappeared. Someone had taken all his stuff. Worse, someone had told the president of Roche that Schadt had directly based his own-written software on the code from the other company, Affymetrix, which was illegal and potentially a huge problem for Roche. Schadt knew he was innocent, but one of his lawyers told him, quite plainly, that the truth is irrelevant: plenty of innocent people go to jail.

On Christmas Eve 1999, Schadt was shopping for presents with his two young kids when his wife phoned to say someone had just telephoned her and needed to talk urgently. Schadt had never heard of the person so he didn't call back and continued shopping with his kids. But the mysterious caller phoned again, this time clarifying that he was from the FBI. Schadt panicked. Why was the FBI after him? Or was this someone pretending to be from the FBI? Tired and scared, he even thought that Affymetrix might have hired a hit man to kill him.

When he got home, it was indeed FBI agents who were waiting for him in a black car outside his house. Schadt was accused of taking the allegedly illegal computer code to the new start-up company.[8] His life became unbearable for months.[9] He saw endless numbers of lawyers. With one, Schadt spent three days going through all the details of the computer codes. The lawyer seemed to take it all in. But at the end, the lawyer politely asked whether algorithms were like logarithms. They're nothing like the same – though the words do rhyme.

Eventually, Schadt met lawyers who could understand computer code, and ultimately it was concluded that he had written his code independently. He became a hero to the academic community, because he had written the computer code simply to do better science and he took on a huge corporation to do so. And then, out of the blue, Schadt's parents called and said he was welcome home again. They had been to a Christian conference where one of the speakers struck a chord with them, leading to them to see a counsellor. They now openly celebrated their son's success.[10]

Schadt's battles – with his family, the military, Affymetrix and the US judiciary – prepared him for the real fight of his life: to establish a new approach in medical research. Whether intentionally or not, Schadt's shorts outfit reminds you of his focus. He's got no time to waste on piffle like thinking about what to wear. Yet, when Schadt visited me on one occasion in 2008, he e-mailed ahead to check if wearing shorts would be OK, or whether he'd need other clothes – perhaps at the evening dinner. Like many successful revolutionaries, he can play at being conventional when needed – he had trained in the air force, after all.

The problem with translating our knowledge into medicine, Schadt and his colleagues argue, is that our effort has just been too simplistic: we've naively focused on finding a causative gene or protein and then a drug to fix it. Perhaps this approach is an inevitable consequence of our brain having evolved to think in terms of one thing leading to the next, or perhaps it's because 'one disease, one gene, one cure' is a straightforward plan readily sold to investors.[11] But our pipeline of new drug development is pretty blocked, because, without mastering the complexity of the system, Schadt argues, it's almost impossible to know what effect a drug will have on something as intricate as the human body.

The side-effects of any new drug, for example, usually only become apparent during a clinical trial because they are so hard to predict in advance. In fact, it's been estimated that about 90 per cent of drugs fail to reach the marketplace because of unexpected side-effects, a direct consequence of the complexity and inter-connectedness of human biology. The thought that most life processes don't work in a straightforward linear way drives most scientists to despair. But here's Schadt's punchline: breathe it all in, embrace complexity, and let's just establish a whole new way of doing things.

Of course, Schadt's advocacy that genes interact in complex ways is not a new idea in itself. In his 1959 BBC Radio lectures, Peter Medawar had said that 'the forms of heredity that can be seen to obey fairly simple rules are not a representative sample of heredity as a whole'.[12] But what Schadt and his like-minded peers are really doing that's new is to establish a way to tackle the complexity; the time is ripe, they say, to navigate us through the fog of genetic interactions and reach medically useful ideas. Science has reduced humanity to a list of genes and components; now to figure out how those elements give rise to the beast itself.

Schadt, and his kindred spirits, argue that what's needed is to reconstruct the underlying networks of interactions between genes causal to traits associated with disease. He thinks that to do this we can sequence DNA, check the functions of cells, measure disease markers – such as levels of sugar and insulin in our blood – and in short obtain an enormous set of information for a huge number of people, to work out which *set of genes* influences each disease or human trait.

The problem is that, even with just ten genes, the number of possible interactions between them is about 10^{18} (a one followed by eighteen zeroes – or a billion billion). And, of course, we don't each have ten genes; we have 25,000. The raw data alone from the sequence of genes in 1,000 individuals amounts to over 10^{12} bytes.[13] Clearly, computing must take centre stage for analysing all the information. The wild-eyed anarchist in a lab coat mixing cells and chemicals is a poor reflection of what's needed for this kind of science. Here, there needs to be multi-disciplinary multi-talented teams that include scientists clicking at computer screens and thinking about abstract algorithms seemingly far removed from the biological processes they're studying. Astronomy, climate change and particle physics have all embraced computationally intensive science long ago; the approach must now be used for studying human health.[14] But before we whole-heartedly nod in agreement, let us recall an allegory with an appropriate cautionary message – a parable from Argentine story-teller Jorge Luis Borges.

There was once an empire where the art of map-making enjoyed the highest reverence. Old maps seemed insufficient, and the Cartographers Guild set out to attain a description of the empire that was truly perfect. But this ultimate ambition – a point-by-point rendition of all the land – only produced a map the same size as the empire itself. The work of the greatest minds culminated in an exact description of the land – *which turned out to be entirely useless.* The perfect map was left discarded, and subsequent generations gave less importance to the art of cartography. 'In the Deserts of the West, still today,' Borges writes, 'there are Tattered Ruins of that Map, inhabited by Animals and Beggars; in all the Land there is no other Relic of the Disciplines of Geography.'[15]

Similarly, a complete and exact simulation of the human body in different states of health and disease may not be a useful ambition – it would be as complex and impenetrable as the human body itself. Schadt and his colleagues aren't concerned, because they aren't seeking to rebuild a human. Their argument is just that we currently have things mapped out too simply and that figuring out the interactions between genes is a depth of detail necessary for developing new drugs. In 2001, the pharmaceutical giant Merck thought similarly and spent $620 million on buying the start-up where Schadt worked. Schadt's plan was to combine conventional laboratory experiments with high-level computational analysis. This would have been difficult in an academic environment but in Merck he could use one of the fastest supercomputers available in the drug industry.

Work in Schadt's biological laboratory determined the extent to which different genes are turned on and off in mice in different states of health and disease. His computer team then used this information to establish which genes are linked together by assessing which genes increased and decreased their activity in concert.[16] They then compared how networks of gene activity altered in mice that had traits associated with obesity, diabetes or hardening of arteries. This complex and iterative process – combining conventional genetic analysis with high-level computation – allowed Schadt and his colleagues to calculate the probabilities of genetic connections and establish causal relationships for disease-associated traits.

With this, they reported the discovery of new genetic networks and sub-networks, with links, edges and hubs – terms more commonly used in describing electrical circuitry. They uncovered a connected group of genes that caused a range of traits such as levels of insulin, glucose, fat and cholesterol – each one being a contributing factor to poor health or disease. They could identify the most important individual genes or proteins that act as nodes or hubs in each genetic circuit. And with that, Merck had new leads for drug development.

Then, in 2008, not long after Schadt's success was clear, Merck announced that it needed to cut 7,200 staff.[17] It was a time when many drug giants were struggling to come up with new products – new drugs based on Schadt's analysis were still only in a developmental stage – and Merck's income was down a third in the quarter leading up to the announcement of job losses. Earlier that year, Merck also paid $58 million in settlement against problems with their block-buster drug for treating arthritis, Vioxx, which allegedly carried an increased risk of heart problems. They were accused of promoting the drug irresponsibly and reportedly had to set aside $4 billion to deal with future claims.[18] As part of the job losses and restructuring, the Seattle site where Schadt was based closed down, and some of its staff moved to research facilities on the East Coast. Schadt and his close colleague Friend didn't want to move – they left Merck and took their big vision with them. But their superfast computers had to stay behind.

Computing technology advances at a breakneck pace: no news there. But biological data is expanding at breakneck pace too, and Schadt's datasets easily outstrip the 1,048,576-row and 16,384-column limit for spreadsheets in Microsoft's Excel.[19] Schadt and Friend couldn't continue without high-level computing. Fortunately, however, they left Merck just as new possibilities were becoming available with companies like Amazon, Google and Microsoft offering on-demand access to their computing infrastructure. These companies provided the relatively bargain-priced way forward they needed.

Schadt continued his mission by establishing – with his colleague Friend – a non-profit organization, Sage Bionetworks, using philanthropic and other funds. Their aim is to now create a common repository of information about people's genes, metabolism and disease from which biological networks can be established and shared by all, and from which drugs can be developed and tested more quickly. The big idea is that, because there is inherent variability in the human population, if only we collect information about enough people then our genetics and traits can be analysed – similar to how Schadt analysed mice – to discover the networks underlying different human diseases.[20] They suggest that this approach implies that we have to abandon many textbook descriptions of disease – because genetic networks rather than single genes are important – dispense with academic cycles of grants and papers, and replace recognition of individual egos with celebrations of teamwork.

The idea that solving complex problems requires teamwork, as well as individual heroes, is a theme throughout the story of compatibility genes: think back to how the early heroes – Dausset, van Rood, Payne and their colleagues – came together in a formative series of international workshops to begin our understanding of human compatibility genes. That early collaboration – the workshops that began in 1964 – triumphed in discovering diversity in human genes. Now, researchers like Schadt argue that a new level of international teamwork is needed to join the parts back together again – to understand how networks of genes give rise to complex human biology.

Nobody is sure how far analysis of biological complexity will take us; as we reach an ever-higher view over our constituent molecules, what will we learn? Is it possible that this approach will help us understand aspects of humanity previously only approached by philosophy or religious belief? The UK's Chief Rabbi, Jonathan Sacks, like many other religious leaders, suggests that science can only put everything together up to a point. He says that humans can do two quite different things. 'One is the ability to break things down into their constituent parts and see how they mesh and interact. The other is the ability to join things together so that they tell a story, and to join people together so that they form relationships. The best example of the first is science, of the second, religion.'[21]

But as we tackle complexity head-on, *à la* Schadt and like-minded biologists, an analysis of networks of genes and traits may allow us to 'join things together' and establish a more complete picture of humanity. Then, depending on how successful science is at putting things together as we move through the twenty-first century, religion might gain in popularity or atheism might spread ceaselessly. These next few steps that scientists take may have sweeping social implications. But for Schadt new medicine is the urgent issue – and how to tackle disease is a debate that's just as fierce as science and religion; because complex analysis of all our variations in genes, traits and diseases isn't the only option on the table.

Others argue that instead we should focus on finding the *rare* genes that underlie extreme versions of a disease. Advocates say this will better indicate where new drugs should be targeted, reasoning that a rare genetic variation that has a big effect (in the few people who have it) can indicate which interactions are important for that disease, even in people without the rare mutation. A powerful example of how a rare human variation has a huge impact comes from a group of people who are very lucky in their resistance to HIV – in a different way from the HIV Controllers.

In the early 1980s, before screening blood for HIV was routine, some haemophiliacs were inadvertently transfused with blood containing the virus. Many died. But there were rare cases in which haemophiliacs had been given HIV-positive blood on several occasions, yet they didn't get AIDS. The tragic mistake of giving people infected blood revealed a new genetic superpower in a few of them.

The mutation that provides this superpower was revealed through some basic research about the virus: specifically, how the virus enters the body's cells. The virus – much smaller than a human cell – first attaches itself to proteins at the surface of human cells before entering them. In 1996, several teams independently reported that one of the proteins that HIV latched on to at the surface of our cells was one called CCR5. Almost immediately afterwards it was discovered that some people have a mutant form of the CCR5 gene in which a small piece of the DNA is missing. People who have inherited two copies of this mutant gene (one from each parent) can't make the normal CCR5 protein. And cells from these people can't be infected with the common form of HIV-1, because it uses the CCR5 protein to latch on to for entering human cells.[22] In 1996, a study following people at risk from HIV found that people with two copies of the mutant gene didn't become sick with AIDS.[23] The new superpower – which allowed some haemophiliacs to resist HIV infection – was in having two copies of a mutant CCR5 gene.[24]

To be clear about how these different results fit together, the study of HIV Controllers set out to discover what gave individuals an ability to stay free from AIDS for some time *after* being infected with HIV. In that case, compatibility genes were the biggest factor – these genes influence how well you can resist illness after infection with the virus. The studies of haemophiliacs, on the other hand, revealed that a mutant form of CCR5 is able to protect *against infection in the first place* – by stopping the virus getting into cells.

The example of CCR5 shows how discovery of a rare mutation does indeed expose a vulnerable aspect of the virus – in this case, its entry into cells. The mutation really is very rare – only about 1 per cent of Europeans have this loss of CCR5 and very few, if any, Africans or Asians do. But the rare mutation reveals a vulnerable aspect of how the virus infects all humans. As a result of this, a range of medicines is based on attacking the docking process by which the virus gets into cells. Drugs have been developed to act as decoys for HIV docking sites or to directly block the proteins used by the virus to latch on to our cells. In future, it may even be possible to manipulate a person's genetics and give them a non-functional version of CCR5. It is – in principle – feasible to treat a person with AIDS by isolating their stem cells, shutting off the CCR5 gene in those cells and then giving them back to the person. This could give anyone the same resistance to HIV as naturally found in those few special haemophiliacs.

There's one individual whose story is probably the most dramatic example you'll ever come across of how one's luck can change.[25] His story is published with the patient remaining anonymous – as required – and it could happen to anybody. This story of this patient began with the unhappy news that he had been infected with HIV. While being treated with standard antiretroviral therapeutic drugs, he was then diagnosed, at age forty, as having cancer as well (specifically, acute myeloid leukaemia). To treat his cancer, the patient had chemotherapy and then needed a stem-cell transplant to replace his cancerous cells.

But instead of transplanting cells from any donor with appropriately matched compatibility genes, the team of medical doctors and scientists took the chance to transplant stem cells from an individual with the genetic variant known to give protection against HIV – that is, from an individual with two copies of the mutant CCR5 gene. Almost unbelievably – but fitting with everything we've discussed – the patient went from having both AIDS *and* cancer to having neither. With one clever stem-cell transfusion, the patient survived two fatal conditions.

So, what's the best route to understanding disease – or path to new medicine: looking for rare genetic variants like mutant CCR5 or screening for common genetic differences like beneficial compatibility genes? The answer: as we've seen – is that both are important. And that's a big reason why funding agencies and philanthropists get pulled in all directions, leaving finances thinly stretched; again, who's to know what's best to do next?

Our genetic complexity also seeds a completely different route to better medicine. Just as we each respond differently to any given infection, we may also respond differently to any given medicine. So, doctors can embrace our individuality – and exploit human complexity – to provide drugs that are personalized to our own genetic needs. And, given that compatibility genes are especially diverse in the human population, it seems pertinent to explore the possibility that these genes could be used to predict how well a specific drug will work or perhaps how bad any side-effects might be. And again a proven example is at hand in the example of HIV – this time in the use of a drug against HIV, abacavir.

Abacavir is potent against HIV but 2–8 per cent of patients react badly to it. A reaction can cause a rash, fever, stomach ache and breathing problems. Treatment has to then stop, because things only get worse and can become life-threatening. Dramatically, in 2002, two teams independently found that having a particular compatibility gene is a strong indicator for who will react badly.[26] Others later confirmed this and the culprit was B*57; in fact, a particular version of B*57. As we've mentioned, different class I compatibility genes are denoted as A, B and C, and versions of each are designated a number such as in B*57. But there are some variants that are very similar to each other. These are formally denoted using additional numbers as B*57:01,

B*57:02, B*57:03 and so on. These 'sub-types' weren't known in the early days of compatibility gene research – they're only easily distinguishable by modern genetic analysis. Importantly here, it turned out that having B*57:01 – and not, say, very similar genes B*57:02 or B*57:03 – correlated with who would react badly to abacavir.

A double-blind, randomized clinical trial tested whether or not screening patients for having B*57:01 would work in predicting who would have bad side-effects. Patients were divided into two groups. In one group everyone was given the drug apart from those patients with B*57:01, and in the other group, absolutely everyone was given the drug as was the normal clinical practice. The result was that the number of people who reacted badly to the drug fell considerably in the screened group.[27] So information about a person's HLA type can be used to reduce the frequency in which a drug has bad side-effects.[28]

Most people would probably accept a doctor's request of a genetic test to ensure a drug won't give them bad side-effects. But fundamentally, why does having HLA-B*57:01 correlate with having side-effects from the HIV drug? Again, it comes down to the ability of HLA proteins to present samples of what's being made inside cells – as peptides – to be checked by immune cells. Cells with B*57:01 and treated with abacavir can potently switch on immune cells, T cells specifically, to kill.[29] Nobody knows how this happens. Perhaps the presence of the drug creates something that gets detected by the immune system as non-self. The drug could do this by triggering a new peptide to be made by cells or by modifying a peptide already made (perhaps by sticking to it).[30] Whatever the precise details are, immune cells activated by B*57:01 cause the damaging side-effects of abacavir.

It is striking that the very same variant of HLA found to be protective against HIV – B*57 – is also the one predictive of side-effects in patients given the HIV drug. Although it seems an unlikely coincidence, it may be just that. It's simply not known whether or not the importance of B*57 in sensitivity to abacavir and in control of HIV is linked in any way beyond the fact that B*57 presents peptides to T cells in both cases. HIV itself plays no role in the side-effects of abacavir; the drug can trigger an immune reaction irrespective of HIV infection.[31] Also, only one sub-type of B*57 triggers the adverse reaction to abacavir, B*57:01, whereas other HLA types can also confer strong protection against HIV, such as B*27 or B*14, or the very closely related variant B*57:03.

The connection between HLA types and side-effects from abacavir explains why people of African or Asian descent almost never react badly to the drug. HLA types aren't evenly distributed among us; we don't just acquire them randomly from the pool of all those possible. Our HLA types are influenced by the diseases our ancestors were exposed to and by the HLA types of people that first populated different parts of the planet. The grand story of human migration and the colonization of our planet is written into the diversity of our HLA genes. And, as a result, Africans or Asians don't often have B*57:01; so they usually have no problem taking abacavir.

It's fascinating to explore this more. Around 150,000 years ago, all modern humans lived in Africa.[32] Genetic evidence for this came during a flurry of activity in the 1980s and '90s from analysing DNA stored in mitochondria, the energy-making parts of cells, and in the male-specific Y chromosome. These two parts of our genome are exceptional in that they are not inherited from both of our parents – only one. The Y chromosome is passed from fathers to sons and mitochondrial DNA is inherited from mothers. So variations in these parts of our DNA are passed on in a relatively simple manner and are easiest to analyse as markers of our ancestry. In 1987, the idea that humans originated in Africa gained genetic backing when an analysis of mitochondrial DNA from many people revealed that they all originated from one woman in Africa, who lived about 200,000 years ago.[33] More recent complex analyses of our genomes have confirmed that humans populated the world by coming out of Africa, and together with archaeology and anthropology, we have sophisticated models for ancient human migration.[34]

It can still be debated exactly where people exited Africa from, if they exited only once, and where humans successfully spread to first, but it's generally accepted that around 100,000 years ago humans successfully left Africa. About 50,000 years ago some reached Europe, and others entered the Americas at least 20,000 years ago. Important to the story of compatibility genes, relatively small groups of founders successfully populated each new territory. It's been suggested, for example, that just hundreds or a few thousand modern humans made it across the Red Sea from East Africa to settle in Yemen and Saudi Arabia.[35] Natural selection then acted on the founders' gene pool as they adapted to the local environment – especially changes in climate, the available food and different types of infections.

Genetic analysis has even indicated that some of the variation in our compatibility genes probably came from us breeding with prehistoric, archaic, humans – Neanderthals and Denisovans.[36] It is possible that the introduction of HLA variants into the modern human population through interbreeding was important in helping increase resistance to local infections. All this together – from human migration to interbreeding – underlies the current geographical structure of our genetic inheritance.

An outcome of this is that Africa retains the greatest genetic diversity in compatibility genes. Within the continent, there's a close correlation between these genes and the different languages spoken – because human migration within Africa over the last 15,000 years has had a significant impact on *both* linguistics and genetics.[37] Then across the world, diversity in our compatibility genes roughly correlates with distance away from Africa, becoming less variable in populations the further away from Africa – because migration to each new territory is seeded by a founding group of people.[38]

In some populations, HLA diversity is particularly limited; among the indigenous people of the Americas, for example, probably because they originated from particularly small founder groups. Brand new versions of HLA-B have relatively recently appeared in some. For example, distinct variants of HLA-B have been found in the Kaingang and Guarani tribes of southern Brazil, and the Waorani people of Ecuador.[39] These versions of HLA-B are likely to be advantageous in fighting particular infections and their impact is perhaps especially important in a population that otherwise has relatively limited variation in HLA. Other rare compatibility genes are found in populations now living separately but related by a common ancestry, such as B*48, which occurs at relatively high frequency amongst Eskimos and other North American Indians, but rarely elsewhere.[40]

There's also a geographical structure to the *combinations* of compatibility genes we each have. That is, many HLA genes occur together more often than would be expected from their individual frequencies. For example, the pairs of genes A*01 with B*08, and A*03 with B*07, both occur more frequently amongst Caucasians than would be expected by chance. A map of HLA types and their combinations in Europe marks out a boundary which corresponds to where the Alps are. Almost certainly this reflects how these mountains have been a barrier to gene flow during early stages of peopling the region.[41]

Overall, the current worldwide map of HLA types is an outcome of natural selection during our battles with infections and the pathways of human migration during the peopling of the world. The implication is that, broadly, our geographic heritage correlates with our susceptibility and resistance to various diseases – and even our response to some drugs.

Many places today are, of course, cosmopolitan, and a database used to keep information on people for potential transplant matches in the UK can reveal precisely how diverse we are.[42] Amazingly, 268,000 people from across the UK are represented by 119,000 different combinations of compatibility genes. This is actually just an underestimation of the true level of our diversity, because the level of precision at which each gene was classified for this analysis was low. Even so, 84,000 combinations of compatibility genes were each represented by just one individual. Single compatibility genes can occur at relatively high frequency, but our complete set of genes is evidently personal: In this analysis, around one in three people were *uniquely* defined by their set of compatibility genes.

Although it remains to be seen exactly how important our individual compatibility genes may be in predicting the appropriate medicine for different diseases, it does seem unlikely that HIV, abacavir and HLA-B*57:01 will be a rare example. More cases like this are likely to emerge as we continue to probe the complexity of diseases. Compatibility genes may also correlate with our responses to vaccines, such as those commonly used for 'flu, polio, measles and rubella.[43] This makes a lot of sense for our differences in class II genes, which encode the HLA proteins found on the specialized immune cells that play a role in initiating the kind of immune response key to successful vaccination. Population-specific vaccines may prove especially effective, though, in truth, we don't yet understand what determines the length of time we remain immune after an infection or a vaccination.

Of course, compatibility genes are not the only genes that can influence our response to drugs. Rituximab, for example, a drug used to treat a certain type of cancer – lymphoma – works best for people with a particular version of another gene in our immune system.[44] In fact, cancer is a prime candidate for treatments to be tailored to an individual's genes. Myeloma, for example, is a cancer of immune cells in the bone marrow – and it is currently incurable. Life expectancies have increased over the last decade, thanks to new drugs, but not everyone responds to everything equally well. Across the world there are differences in treatments – the timing, combinations and doses of different drugs used in combination with stem-cell transplants all vary considerably. Much is decided on an ad hoc basis. Like many cancer treatments, personalized regimens are the norm – but the decisions are based on local expertise, far from being standardized.

The genetic make-up of myelomas from different people has been analysed and no single genetic factor causes this cancer.[45] In fact, each myeloma cell has, on average, tens of genetic differences from the patient's normal cells. Some mutations are common, including some involved in processes targeted by drugs already available. But a new opportunity has come from genetic analysis of myeloma; once again, instead of being defeated by the complexity, we could exploit it. Patients could have their cancer cells analysed genetically so that the appropriate treatment could be selected without wasting time testing drugs by trial and error – avoiding side-effects from drugs that can't help. In this way, even though we don't understand fully how the mutations combine to make a cell cancerous, we can just exploit the fact that it's complicated to improve treatment.

It's just an idea: it remains to be clinically proven. But there are many clinicians and scientists advocating that such personalized (or stratified) medicine should become a reality in the very near future. Technology for analysing genes currently improves about fourfold each year, and, if that continues, we'll have sequenced the genomes of a million different people by 2016. That will be enough data to validate all kinds of specific genetic diagnostics. But there's still a problem. One reason why this is not guaranteed to work out is that there can be great variety in the tumour cells themselves – even in a single patient. Even within one person, individual cancer cells can vary in their drug sensitivity. This situation is similar to what we saw with HIV: a highly variable enemy is more difficult to attack.

Viruses and tumours do something else that's a problem – they actively thwart our defences. One way they do this is by trying to prevent our compatibility genes from working. It's a battle; our immune system fights back by checking if compatibility genes have been interfered with. This involves a whole other function of our compatibility genes, a different way of looking at the immune system, and another set of immune genes that are also extremely diverse among us – in fact, they are probably only second to compatibility genes in how variable they are from person to person. This next piece of the canvas – hard-won by new heroes – reveals how compatibility genes can work in the exact *opposite* way to what we've discussed so far. Breathe it all in, embrace the complexity.

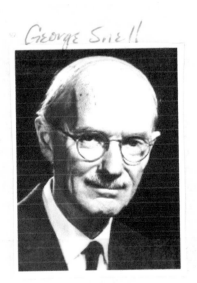

George Snell

7

Missing Self

Klas Kärre would later chair the committee that decides the Nobel Prize in Physiology or Medicine, but in 1981, while writing his PhD thesis, he was less secure. Trying to summarize his observations in the last chapter of his thesis, he was puzzled by some data that didn't seem consistent with the prevailing ideas about how the immune system worked. Kärre – described by his PhD supervisor, Rolf Kiessling, as soft-spoken, eloquent and slightly absent-minded[1] – thought about the problem a lot. Others had come across the same discrepancies but just didn't think them particularly important. What often distinguishes the great from the everyday scientists is their ability to think lucidly about observations that don't fit with contemporary paradigms. As Leonard Cohen sings, 'There is a crack in everything, that's how the light gets in.'[2]

Once again, experiments in transplantation were at the heart of the matter. Recall that a transplant is rejected whenever it has proteins detected as non-self which cause an immune attack. But there was an exception to this rule – first observed in the 1950s by George Snell, working in the Jackson Laboratory, Maine, USA, a small, independent non-profit research institution. He discovered a situation in which transplants would be rejected even when they didn't have non-self proteins.

To understand the mystery – to think about it deeply like Kärre did – we need to consider the genetics of the inbred mice used in Snell's experiments. Inbred mice are obtained by successive breeding between siblings (or parents and their offspring) over long periods.[3] Offspring from two different types of inbred mice are called the F1 hybrid. Not the cutest of baby names, it stands for *Filial* 1 hybrid and is a widely used genetic term to describe offspring from different strains of animals or plants. For example, a mule is the F1 hybrid of a male donkey and a female horse. That is, a mule came about when a donkey and horse mated rather than being a species that evolved through gradual changes in an ancestor of all three animals.

The importance of inbreeding here is that all the mice from one inbred population have identical compatibility genes – the normal diversity being wiped out by the inbreeding. Usually, there are different compatibility genes on each strand in the double-helix shape of our DNA. On one strand of the helix there are genes inherited from the mother and on the other strand there are genes from the father. This gives us, for example, two versions of the HLA-A gene. But, because inbred strains of mice have the same compatibility genes on each strand of their DNA, there's no variation in what they pass on to their children. And – crucial to the transplantation mystery – F1 hybrids inherit all of the compatibility genes found in their parents. So F1 hybrids should be able to accept transplanted tissue from either parent.

But here's the mystery: Snell found this to be true for skin or organs like kidneys – these can be successfully transplanted from parents to an F1 hybrid – but transplants of bone marrow are rejected nonetheless. Why was bone marrow rejected? It's a violation of the basic rule for transplantation, because the parents' cells do not have non-self compatibility genes.[4] It was a crack in our understanding through which a whole other aspect of our immune system would be uncovered – starting with the discovery of a new type of cell.

In 1971, scientists at the State University of New York, Buffalo, USA, glimpsed that a new immune cell could be responsible for the rejection of bone-marrow transplants.[5] They found that mice with their thymus surgically removed would still reject bone marrow. Since T cells need the thymus to develop properly, this indicated that something other than these immune cells was responsible for the transplant rejection. But it took several more years for clearer progress to be made in solving the transplantation mystery. What turned out to be crucial were experiments by scientists tackling an entirely different problem, nothing to do with F1 hybrids or transplantation, but rather with cancer.

During the early to mid-1970s, many teams of researchers across the globe were performing experiments to compare how well diseased cells – such as cancer cells – could be killed by immune cells taken from different people (or different animals). They would test, for example, how well immune cells taken from different patients with leukaemia could kill cancer cells, in comparison with immune cells taken from healthy people. The thinking was that leukaemia patients would have immune cells activated to be efficient killers because of their exposure to leukaemic cells, while immune cells from healthy people should not be able to kill cancer cells – they would serve as the 'blank' control sample. But it was often found that immune cells from healthy people could, in fact, kill cancerous cells.

Even more surprising, cancer cells could be killed by a person's white blood cells even when their T cells – the type of cell everyone thought was responsible for killing cancer cells – were deliberately removed. Most scientists took this as merely an inconvenient 'background' killing, likely caused by some inaccuracy in the way that killing was measured. A few people thought that there could be an odd type of T cell left behind after most had been removed. Hardly anybody considered that there could be an altogether new type of cell responsible for killing cancer cells.

Most teams simply ploughed on regardless – trying not to get distracted by the 'background' problem. Some researchers found ways to circumvent the issue – by only using blood from donors whose cells happened to be particularly weak at killing the cancer cells being studied. In effect, they were exploiting the diversity in immune responses to get rid of the 'background' problem. They set up their experiments so that the results would fit with contemporary ideas about what *should* happen. It seems erroneous in hindsight, but in fact it's not that they were being particularly bad scientists; this kind of blinkered view is often necessary. When a computer crashes, who thinks it's worth spending the rest of the day trying to figure out precisely what happened? We all just swear a bit, try 'Ctrl + Alt + Delete' and then just turn the computer off and on again to keep moving. It's just extremely hard to know when an unexpected result has something important at its root. There's always a rush to new knowledge – and to get a PhD, next job, or grant – and who's got the time to hang about wondering why a computer crashed, or why there's an irritating background signal coming from the blank control?

To realize that something interesting hid in the 'background' took a certain attitude. Months or years of hard work could be wasted if some boring technical problem is all that's uncovered. A scientist's life isn't at stake in the same way as when an astronaut accepts the danger of space flight, but you still need something of the right stuff to take on and solve a scientific mystery. The breakthrough that solved the 'background' problem – and in turn, the transplantation mystery – came from two pioneers working independently; Ronald Herberman at the US National Cancer Institute and Rolf Kiessling in Stockholm, Sweden.[6]

In 1970, at the age of twenty-two, Kiessling had begun his doctoral studies at the Karolinska Institute, Stockholm, a renowned hub for studying immune responses to tumours. His plan was to find out how well mouse T cells could kill a particular tumour cell (called YAC-1). It was a fortuitous choice, because YAC-1 is killed especially well by the immune cell responsible for the 'background' killing; so the 'background' killing was particularly high, harder to ignore. Kiessling realized that the tumour cells were being killed by cells other than T cells and he named them Natural Killer (NK) cells.[7] NK cells are, in fact, especially good at attacking cancer cells – and also some types of virus-infected cells. There are about 1,000 of them in every drop of your blood, and each is capable of killing around twelve cancer cells. But after Kiessling published his paper, he saw Herberman's report on the same new immune cell. So many people participate in modern science that it's hard for anyone to make an important discovery in the way they dreamed they would – on their own. Rather than being relieved that his findings had been confirmed immediately, Kiessling was frustrated by the competition.[8]

For a decade, Kiessling continued studying NK cells but then, in the mid-1980s, he decided to change direction entirely. He simply wanted to try another area of research and he wanted to work on something closer to human disease.[9] He stopped going to scientific meetings on NK cells and, in 1986, he moved to Ethiopia to work on leprosy (known as Hansen's disease in the US). He decided that he should study the immune response against the bacteria that cause leprosy, thinking this might indicate a way to vaccinate against the disease. Arguably, it was a bad career move. He had his reputation sealed for ever among scientists studying NK cells and was unknown in the world of leprosy research.[10] The irony is that it wouldn't be long before NK cell research did become relevant to human diseases – as our understanding of these cells deepened. Kiessling has no regrets and says his time in Africa was one of the most exciting periods in his life.[11] He could return to conferences about NK cells at any time – where he would be welcomed, revered even – but, talking to me in 2011, he said, 'I would hate that – turning up like some kind of dinosaur.'[12]

Shortly before Kiessling left for Africa, in 1985, the other discoverer of NK cells, Herberman, became the founding director of the University of Pittsburgh Cancer Institute.[13] He successfully directed the institute for almost twenty-four years but towards the end of his tenure, in 2008, he became the centre of a national controversy when he issued a statement to advise everyone in the Cancer Institute that they should reduce their use of mobile phones. He issued a two-page memorandum which included advice to not allow children to use a mobile – except for emergencies – and to avoid carrying one on your body at all times. The multi-billion-dollar phone industry wasn't happy; and the furore was reported in national and international newspapers, magazines and on TV news stations. Herberman defended himself, saying that we shouldn't wait for a definitive study to come out, but should err on the side of caution.[14] Though he had published more than 700 scientific papers and discovered nothing less than a new type of cell, his stance on mobile phone use garnered him the most public attention by far.

Herberman's and Kiessling's discovery of a new immune cell was not immediately hailed as a breakthrough because, at the time, technology for discriminating between different types of cells was relatively primitive. And it took another four years for the equivalent cells to be identified in humans. Human NK cells looked very different to T cells when viewed under a microscope: much more speckled, or, to use the technical term, more granular.[15] Their speckled appearance easily stood out – and this was formative in everyone agreeing that NK cells really were a new type of immune cell.[16]

The discovery of NK cells solved the transplantation mystery; these immune cells were responsible for the rejection of bone-marrow transplants (in F1 hybrids). The killer had been identified – but what was their motive? As one enigma unravelled another opened up: what caused the NK cells to attack transplanted bone marrow? Did they use a similar strategy to T cells to detect disease – self/non-self – or did they have an entirely different battle-plan? NK cells could not have evolved to detect transplanted bone marrow because that would never happen naturally. But there had to be a clue in the transplantation mystery as to how NK cells really worked – because the way that NK cells detect diseased cells must cause them to attack transplanted bone marrow.

Another clue to how NK cells worked was that some tumour cells, readily killed by these immune cells, actually lacked proteins encoded by compatibility genes – the HLA proteins. Most people took this to mean that NK cells must recognize some signature of disease which had nothing to do with HLA. As a result, research programmes around the world focused on finding something other than HLA proteins on transplanted cells that would be detected by NK cells. But the young Swedish PhD student Kärre came up with a different idea.

For the final sentence of his PhD thesis, Kärre wanted to write down the strategy used by NK cells to detect signs of disease in other cells.[17] Focusing on overarching principles about how the immune system works is reminiscent of Burnet's ambition to discover the grand unified theory of immunology, but Kärre's approach was more pragmatic. Kärre collated all the available data – his own as well as everything he could read about – and then set about trying to summarize them. This was different from the way Burnet thought in more abstract terms about how an immune system *could* work: Kärre simply listed all the situations in which NK cells were good at killing diseased cells to see if he could fathom a common denominator.[18]

He had begun his journey to this point because of one crucial phone call that went unanswered. In 1975, at age twenty-one, while in his second year of studies to become a medical doctor, he read that George Klein, the head of the Tumour Biology Research, was looking for someone to help in their research. At his interview, Kärre began to tell Klein all about himself, but Klein interrupted to tell him that none of that was important: 'What I need to know is when can you start?'[19]

Kärre said he could start the next day, which got him the job, and immediately Klein tried to phone the researcher he had in mind to work with Kärre, but he wasn't around. Flustered, Klein just called someone else and arranged for them instead to work with Kärre. A tiny moment on which great things hinged; this second researcher was Kiessling – and that's how Kärre got to work on the newly discovered NK cells.[20]

After years of studying these new cells, it was during a stay at his soon-to-be parents-in-law – trying to finish his PhD thesis – that Kärre had an epiphany. It occurred to him that cells readily killed by NK cells were often resistant to killing by T cells, and vice-versa. Thinking about the problem in this way, he realized that T cells only killed cells that have proteins encoded by compatibility genes, while NK cells were best at killing cells in which these proteins were *absent*. His stroke of genius was to recognize that the very fact these proteins were *not* there might be the signal NK cells used to detect that something was wrong.

The unlikely source of inspiration for Kärre's revelation was a defence strategy used by the Swedish navy.[21] The navy command had become worried about the presence of foreign submarines entering their waters and decided that a low-cost option for surveillance would be to educate local fishermen to keep an eye out for them. Their initial plan was to give fishermen leaflets showing silhouettes of the submarines they should look out for. Anybody who saw a submarine that looked like one in the leaflet should alert the navy. But there were all kinds of possible submarines, and anybody seeing one would have to go through several pages to check for a match. Realizing that this was cumbersome, the navy came up with a second plan of issuing fishermen with one single page showing three submarines – the Swedish ones – along with the instruction that if they saw a submarine that was *not* one of those pictured then they should alert the navy. Rather than directly looking for something foreign, the best strategy was to check for what was expected and, if it wasn't that, then it should be considered a problem.

Kärre realized the navy strategy applied to NK cells. Rather than directly looking for unexpected molecules as a signature of disease, NK cells could check for proteins that are normally on cells as a sign of health. Compatibility genes are at the centre of this. It is the proteins that they encode for – the HLA proteins – that is precisely what is checked for. Nearly all cells in your body have HLA proteins at their surface – to allow them to be checked by T cells – so any cell that lacks these proteins at the surface must be abnormal in some way. Indeed, many cancer cells contain mutations that cause them to lack HLA proteins at their surface – presumably helping the cancerous cell avoid detection by T cells. And HIV, for example, has its own way of stopping HLA proteins doing their job properly.[22] NK cells defend against this – by noticing whether HLA proteins are missing. It was the epiphany that gave Kärre the grand ending he wanted for his PhD thesis: the immune system searches for things that should not be in your body *and* checks for the presence of normal proteins that should be there.

Back again to the transplantation mystery. Recall that we got to the point where (F1 hybrid) NK cells were discovered to attack bone-marrow transplants from their parents, but the new problem was in understanding why. The situation was mysterious, because an F1 hybrid inherits all of Mum and Dad's compatibility genes, so there is nothing that could be detected as non-self to trigger an immune reaction against the transplant. Kärre's epiphany provided the solution: when bone-marrow cells from one parent – say Mum's cells – are transplanted, they only have half the set of compatibility genes that the F1 hybrid has – Mum's but not Dad's. So some proteins are *missing* in the transplanted cells; NK cells, abundant in bone marrow, detect this loss of protein – and attack.

No longer thinking this should just be one sentence in his PhD thesis, Kärre thought to announce his idea in his thesis title. Kiessling, his supervisor, considered it unwise, because this was still merely an unproven hypothesis. Kiessling and Kärre were similar in age and openly criticized each other's opinions. This was important to their success: heated, back-and-forth banter is often necessary for thoughts to crystallize. Kärre was awarded his PhD in 1981, but his big idea was indeed left out of his thesis title. It didn't really matter, because, despite being the culmination of many years' hard work, a PhD thesis is rarely read by anyone anyway.

Eventually, Kärre's hypothesis got the wider attention it deserved when, aged thirty, he was one of the youngest presenters at the second-ever NK Cell Workshop, held near Detroit in 1984. Although the audience thought his new idea interesting, it was far from being instantly accepted. Most delegates were sceptical – and when scientists politely say in public that they are sceptical, they'll be clearer in the bar and say they think it's bullshit.

Kärre thought to himself that, if it turned out that he was wrong, he would leave scientific research and embrace a clinical career instead.[23] Resistance in the community wasn't simply inertia against anything new; scientists were sceptical because there was some data that didn't seem consistent with Kärre's idea. For example, some cells could be killed by NK cells even when they had MHC proteins present, so it wasn't clear-cut that *only* those without them were killed. At least initially, other views about NK cells seemed equally plausible: maybe NK cells were able to recognize some other protein – one that remained to be discovered – as a sign of disease.

But the biggest problem with acceptance of Kärre's idea was that it seemed to suggest something completely opposite to what was already known about these proteins. The proteins encoded by compatibility genes were established as being important for *activating* immune cells – capable of switching on T cells to attack. Now, they were being proposed as also being able to *turn off* immune cells – albeit different immune cells; NK cells. One scientist likened the idea to somebody saying you could play the Beatles backwards and still get meaningful lyrics.[24]

In 1986, two years after Kärre first presented his idea at the Detroit meeting, he found that mouse tumour cells deliberately chosen to lack MHC proteins were indeed efficiently killed by NK cells.[25] With this result, Kärre was sure that his idea couldn't be entirely wrong. A few years later, in 1990, he published a hugely influential article with his first doctoral student, Hans-Gustaf Ljunggren, elaborating on the idea and naming it the 'missing self' hypothesis.[26] Good names are important – the Big Bang is another example. Art also helped; the cover to the journal featuring the 'missing self' hypothesis showed a woman looking into a large mirror with her reflection absent.

As Kärre's idea gained traction, attention shifted to the problem of *how* immune cells could know when a normal molecule was missing on another cell. One way this could work would be if NK cells had receptor proteins on their surface that stop NK cells from killing whenever they bind to MHC protein on another cell. In this way, when an NK cell touches another cell that has MHC proteins, the NK cell receives a signal to *not* kill. But if MHC proteins are missing on any cell, the NK cell receptor proteins have nothing to interact with – the brake signal is lost and the NK cell delivers its kiss of death. This seemed the simplest way in which NK cells could survey other cells for the presence of a normal self protein – but the question was whether or not such a receptor really existed; the search was on for the missing 'missing self' receptor.[27]

Once again, the problem was solved out of left field. Without thinking about the 'missing self' hypothesis at all, Wayne Yokoyama – born in Hawaii – had been working at the Washington University School of Medicine, St Louis, to identify new receptor proteins on immune cells and in 1989 he found one that he called A1.[28] It was later renamed Ly49 and Wayne's wife, Lynn Yokoyama, truly believes he named it after her. In truth, it's named as the forty-ninth member in the Ly family of proteins that share certain chemical features.[29] Yokoyama found out that Ly49 came in many different forms. He hadn't any clue that Ly49 would turn out to be central to Kärre's 'missing self' hypothesis but he was confident that he was on to something important – because he thought that the protein's variability must mean something interesting.

Yokoyama – who has a zen-like quality of always seeming calm and relaxed – had initially been turned on to medical research through a high school project he did.[30] Yokoyama's father had died when he was fourteen, and his school teacher mentored and supported him through the difficult times that followed, later helping him obtain a summer placement at the hospital where Hawaii's first kidney transplant between twins had just happened.[31] Aged seventeen, Yokoyama worked with doctors who were beginning to optimize transplantation success using tests that had recently been established by the early pioneers of HLA – those we met in Chapter 3. The population of Hawaii is exceptionally diverse, and Yokoyama could see patterns in blood reactivity when he ordered his results according to each individual's ethnicity. He could see that this could have a major impact in medical transplantation and decided he should become a medical doctor.[32]

Later in life, when it became clear that part of the job as a medic is to ask patients intimate details about issues such as their sex life, he decided that his place was in the lab.

After working at the NIH, Yokoyama earned a faculty position in University of California San Francisco (UCSF) and decided to focus his new lab on the protein he had recently discovered, Ly49. At that point, the protein could have had any role at all in the body. But he found out that the Ly49 gene was positioned close to another gene already known to be active in NK cells, and that gave him a clue that he should look at those cells. By separating NK cells according to whether or not they had Ly49, he found out that NK cells which lacked Ly49 killed other cells especially well. This indicated that the presence of the Ly49 protein on NK cells worked to *prevent* them killing.

By comparing how well NK cells could kill different types of tumour cells, it was eventually worked out that the Ly49 receptor turned off the NK cell killing machinery when it bound to MHC proteins on another cell in contact. If MHC proteins were missing on a cell in contact with an NK cell, the signal from Ly49 to 'switch-off' gets lost and the NK cell delivers its lethal hit.[33] Yokoyama had identified the molecular process that lets the immune system search for 'missing self' – through a receptor protein that checks for presence of MHC proteins on other cells. Yokoyama's discovery vindicated Kärre's original idea about NK cells, and both scientists became well known as a result. In 2009, Kärre gained the prestigious position of chairing the committee that decides who wins the Nobel Prize for Medicine and Physiology.[34] He doesn't like to talk about it; the committee conducts its work in high secrecy, for reasons that are obvious, given the gossip we're about to come across.

Yokoyama's discovery was in mice. It was important to find out whether or not NK cells worked the same way in humans; the next race was to find the equivalent of Ly49 in us. Research teams searched for a protein that looked like Ly49 on human NK cells – or a gene that encoded for one. Many years passed, and the human equivalent simply couldn't be found. The question arose: could a defence strategy as elegant as the search for 'missing self' only be used by rodents?

Then – as we've seen happen before – two teams reported the

solution at the same time.[35] But gossip circulated soon after to suggest that one of the team's leaders had listened to a lecture by the other – and from that had gained a vital clue that they had then used to identify the receptor. It could well be a rumour without merit, but I mention it, not to take anything away from the achievement of the scientists involved, but to show that gossip circulates in science probably no differently to the banter that goes on in art, music, literature or any other area of human achievement. Tales like this exist for many big discoveries – and even small ones where establishing priority has no impact anyway.

The clue that one scientist may or may not have gained from the other was the protein's type (and its chemistry at one end). It was crucial information, because the human version of Ly49 was not much like mouse Ly49; for years, everybody had been looking for something that would be similar to mouse Ly49, but the human version turned out to be altogether different. The human counterpart to mouse Ly49 has very different chemical features – and is part of the so-called immunoglobulin family of proteins, which gives them their cumbersome name of Killer Immunoglobulin-like Receptors, or KIR.

KIR

Important processes for life usually evolved in a common ancestor to mice and humans. That is why genes and proteins are often very similar in both species. But here, different kinds of protein operate an identical aspect of the immune system. The implication is that the strategy of looking for missing self as a signature of disease is useful to many species – but the process to make it work has evolved relatively recently so that it is different in mice and men.

This difference – of mice and men – is important because mice are commonly used for testing and developing new medicines; they're relatively easy to keep and breed fast, and a lot of technology has been developed around mice so that, for example, it's easy to genetically manipulate them. I write this as fact – not as an advocate for animal experiments, which is a complex issue that needs a separate discussion. In support of using mice for medical research – as opposed to another animal – it's often quoted that the genomes of all mammals are remarkably similar. Precise details depend on what's compared; roughly 99 per cent of mouse genes have a human counterpart, each being around 85 per cent similar on average. However, there's no mouse version of AIDS or many other human diseases. And the different kinds of NK cell receptors used to search for 'missing self' are a good example of where mouse and human immune systems differ. A drug designed to block these receptors on human NK cells, for example, cannot be tested in mice because they simply don't have that protein for the drug to act on. This is not an academic point; it's a major problem for testing new medicine.

Such a drug – to block the NK cell's 'switch-off' receptors – is, for example, in development at the French company InnatePharma (and licensed to the pharma giant Bristol-Myers Squibb). The idea is to unleash NK cells so they may be able to kill cancer cells, or other diseased cells, more effectively than normal. To test the drug in mice, receptors from human NK cells have to be genetically added to the animals. Technically it's not that difficult to do this – scientists have been shuffling genes between species for a long time now – but it's easy to see how this approach soon gets fiddly. Because, when adding the human NK cell receptors to mice, the human MHC proteins they bind to should also be genetically added – and then how much more besides?[36]

A common approach is to start with a mouse that has been mutated to lack much of its immune system and then add human genes or stem cells to create so-called humanized mice. Like 'missing self' and 'The Big Bang', the name 'humanized mice' is evocative, and this truly is as close to creating Frankenstein's monster as medical science gets. For now, it seems impossible that any level of higher-order human brain functions could be reconstituted in an animal, but on the other hand we have no idea how far this could go. A more immediate concern – pertinent to the story of compatibility genes – is that even in the most human of humanized mice, our *diversity* is missing.

Like the HLA proteins they detect, our NK cell receptors are highly variable. Individual KIR genes vary less than our HLA genes, but there's an altogether different kind of disparity among us for these NK cell genes. Variation in HLA genes is huge – as we've seen – but at least the number of them is fixed. On the other hand, KIR genes – those that encode the NK cell receptor proteins – also differ in the number we each have. This means that not only can we inherit different versions of these genes, but also large chunks of genetic code for

NK cell receptors are present or absent in each of us. Although the effect this has on our immune system isn't fully understood, it is already clear that our inheritance of KIR genes influences our susceptibility and resistance to disease, especially in combination with specific compatibility genes – as first discovered in 2004 for hepatitis C.[37]

Around one in five people infected with hepatitis C can clear the virus on their own. For others – 170 million people worldwide – the infection persists and can cause major liver damage. Many factors influence what happens after infection – such as the particular strain of the virus. A mutation in an immune-system gene called IL28B has an especially strong impact on clearance of virus – which helps account for different success rates in treating patients from European or African-American ancestry.[38] Compatibility genes also influence our response – as we've seen for all kinds of different diseases – but the twist here is that compatibility genes do not on their own correlate with who fares better or worse with hepatitis C; rather a particular *combination* of HLA and KIR genes seems to help.[39]

Unfortunately, it's not understood why – this is at a frontier of our knowledge about compatibility genes. The situation is complicated, because some of our KIR genes encode the receptors that we've discussed – those that switch off NK cells when seeing HLA proteins on other cells, enabling the search for 'missing self' as a sign of disease. But there are other versions of these receptors that do the opposite; some KIR genes encode for proteins that signal to switch *on* NK cells rather than deactivate them. And guess what: these genes also vary considerably between us.

The way that these activating versions of NK cell receptors help fight disease remains to be discovered. One possibility is that these receptors can recognize decoy versions of HLA proteins made by viruses as they try to thwart our immune defences. A plausible scenario runs as follows: a virus infects a cell and avoids detection by T cells by stopping our HLA proteins from working properly. NK cells should be able to detect the loss of HLA proteins according to the 'missing self' hypothesis – they can detect that HLA proteins are missing from the surface of the infected cells. But this is a war; and so the virus makes its own lookalike HLA protein, which it hopes will fool the NK cells. Still, the viral decoy isn't quite the genuine article, and perhaps the NK cell's activating receptors can spot the difference. That way, the infected cell would get detected and killed after all. Plausible – but nobody knows if this is what really happens.[40] It's also possible that these activating receptors aren't primarily for our defence against disease at all; they could play a different role in our body, such as in pregnancy – something we'll come back to later.

Combinations of compatibility genes and NK cell genes have also been linked with our response to HIV. But here the findings are, in short, bewildering. For HIV, activating *as well as* inhibitory NK cell receptors – in combination with the HLA proteins they bind to – can be protective.[41] There's also evidence that the virus adapts according to the NK cell receptor genes that a person has – presumably to avoid detection in that person.[42] We can't explain what is going on in detail, other than to say that NK cells play some role in killing cells infected with HIV. There's a crack in everything.

Recall that scientists were initially sceptical about the 'missing self' hypothesis because some cancerous cells were killed by NK cells even when they had MHC proteins working normally. This stands up to scrutiny and in fact is a good example of how hard it is to piece together the rules that govern a biological system – because there are often exceptions. We now understand that detection of 'missing self' is just *one way* by which NK cells can detect diseased cells. There are other ways too. NK cells also attack cells that are stressed. Not 'stressed' in the everyday sense of the word – an individual cell can't feel an emotional strain – but cells do have a way to sense when something is wrong inside and can undergo what's called a stress response.

It's common knowledge that too much UV light is bad for skin – because UV light can damage DNA. When that happens, cells detect the broken DNA inside them and respond – and that's what is meant by a cell responding to being stressed. As part of this stress response, the cell attempts to repair its DNA but also the damaged cell will put up at its surface certain proteins that are not normally found on healthy cells but appear only when a cell is stressed. By putting these special proteins on its surface a cell can indicate to neighbouring cells that it's damaged. NK cells detect these stress-induced proteins and by doing so they know when another cell is damaged or 'stressed' – and they can kill them. So, as well as detecting missing self as a sign of trouble, NK cells also detect 'induced self' by looking for a protein not normally found on cells but one that appears when a cell knows it's in trouble. NK cells – and probably all other types of immune cells – are capable of detecting disease through several different strategies.[43] Our immune system works in myriad ways – and compatibility genes play a central role.

It has taken over five decades since HLA was discovered to reach this level of understanding of our immune system – and seven chapters of this book to describe. And, broadly, scientists are in agreement with the story so far. What comes next, however, is far more contentious. In the final part of this book, we will discuss the evidence that our compatibility genes – undoubtedly central to how our immune system works – also influence the way we choose lovers and the success of pregnancies, perhaps even the wiring of our brains. If so, there are two ways of viewing this. First, our bodies may just happen to reuse the same genes and proteins to do different things. The alternative is that these different aspects of humanity are intimately linked. And my view is that the latter is more likely to be true: that compatibility genes play a role in defence against disease and reproduction because these two essentials of life are fundamentally connected.

PART THREE

The Overarching System

8

Sex and Smelly T-shirts

Medawar's experiments in transplantation showed that our bodies can distinguish our own cells from those of other people through differences in compatibility genes. At the time, everyone was in agreement that these genes could not have evolved merely to make transplantation difficult, because it's such an unnatural situation. The foremost function of these genes – as discovered later – is in the immune system. But the ability of these genes to cause problems in transplantation may not be so far removed from one of their real roles after all, because these genes could indeed mark our identity – and influence interpersonal compatibility – through our sense of smell.

Rimmel begins his bestseller *The Book of Perfumes*, published in 1864, five years after Darwin's *On the Origin of Species*: 'Among the many enjoyments provided for us by bountiful Nature, there are few more delicate and, at the same time, more keen than those derived from the sense of smell.'[1] Yet around 150 years later – while the details of Darwinian evolution have been mined extensively – we understand relatively little about smell. Luca Turin, a scientist and perfumer, reveals in his popular book published in 2006, *The Secret of Scent*: 'The secret is this: though we now know almost everything there is to know about molecules, we don't know *how our nose reads them*.'[2]

An unofficial analysis of one perfume – *Beyond Paradise* by Estée Lauder – revealed that it contained about 400 different molecules.[3] We know something about how our nose detects these chemicals, using thousands of specialized receptors which take up around 3 per cent of the human genome, but we understand precious little about how our brain uses the information to give us the perception of a smell and in turn, subconsciously, or consciously, influence our behaviour.

Turin suggests that there's been little investment for research into smell because the practical benefit isn't as obvious as, say, medicine and technology.[4] There's been far more research – Turin says – to understand our senses of vision and hearing because they are considered more important, life being so much worse if you lose them. My own view is that we understand little about smell because it's just so difficult to study. Colours can be characterized by wavelengths of light; shapes can be represented by mathematical equations; sound is stored in digital form in every download; but how do you describe the smell of vanilla?

We don't even have the language to depict a smell in the way that a visual picture, for example, is easily described. Writers portray smells in metaphors or analogies; we certainly can't *calculate* how any molecule smells. Computers can't predict a perfect-smelling concoction of molecules, and perfumes are made by experts literally just following their nose. Most problematic of all, for the science of smell, human responses to smells can only be assessed with woolly scoring systems that are hard to interpret unambiguously. And, as we will see, this causes huge controversy.

In 1994, undeterred by these problems in studying smell, Claus Wedekind, a Swiss zoologist then working at the University of Bern, Switzerland, set up a fascinating experiment. He asked women to rank different men's T-shirts as to how sexy or pleasant they smelt, aiming to find out whether or not their preferences corresponded to how similar or dissimilar compatibility genes were between the men wearing the T-shirts and the women smelling them. Wedekind didn't arrive at this experiment with any background in immunology. Instead, he had been thinking about how animals and people assess potential mates – as in how female peacocks assess the display of a male's feathers.

He had been studying bumps called tubercles found on male fish, thought to indicate an individual's breeding fitness to females – exactly like a peacock's feathers. He realized that it wasn't clear what the female fish were assessing about tubercles – their number or size, for example – and, most importantly, what was actually being indicated by tubercles that related to being a good partner for breeding. He also realized (as others did) that the system seemed like it could be open to cheating: animals could display a desirable trait, like many large tubercles or beautiful feathers, without having any qualities that females could actually benefit from – they could be faking it.

To study this, Wedekind used a mathematical simulation of what would happen if males cheated and predicted situations in which honesty would win out in the long term. The bottom line was that cheaters wouldn't win as long as genes that directly influence survival could be sensed with little effort. He then read about research indicating that mice could sense each other's immune-system genes by smell – which seemed to fit his theoretical ideas for how mate selection should work.

Although the idea that compatibility genes can be a distinguishing mark of our individuality goes right back to Peter Medawar's discoveries in the 1950s, Medawar never entertained the possibility that humans or animals could actually sense an individual's compatibility genes.[5] It took until the early 1970s for this idea to be taken seriously;[6] when Jeanette Boyse, working in a research team led by her British-born husband Ted Boyse at the Memorial Sloan-Kettering Cancer Centre in New York, happened to notice that mice she was breeding seemed to prefer to mate with specific other mice.[7] The husband and wife team wondered if these preferences might correlate with compatibility genes.

Lewis Thomas, a well-known scientist and prominent essayist of the time who headed the New York institute where the Boyses worked, theoretically considered that compatibility genes could give individuals a particular scent. In his essay 'A fear of pheromones', published in his 1974 collection *Lives of the Cell*, he explicitly questioned whether or not dogs might be able to sniff out humans according to their compatibility genes.[8] Actually, we still don't really know the answer to that: dogs can have sixty times as many smell receptors as humans, and some can reportedly detect the scent of a person from a week-old fingerprint, but we know little about how this works.

Thomas came to this idea not by directly observing the mating preferences of mice but in thinking about disparate observations made by others in the early 1970s. One rather bizarre source of inspiration was the tale of a loner living on an island who made the discovery that 'by taking the dry weight of the hairs trapped by his electric razor every day, that his beard grew much more rapidly each time he returned to the mainland and encountered girls.'[9] Thomas took the anecdote – published anonymously[10] – as evidence that we are affected by the presence of others in subtle ways. Another observation reported at the time was the spontaneous synchronization of menstrual cycles for women living together. Thomas saw this to also signify a new-found interpersonal communication – and perhaps something that worked through odours.[11] Forty years on, menstrual synchronization remains controversial. Although 80 per cent of women believe it happens, there still isn't agreement amongst scientists whether or not it occurs, never mind understanding how it works.[12]

Thinking about these phenomena, Thomas, as well as others, realized that if people or animals could sense each other in some way – perhaps by smell – there had to be a fixed genetic component involved, because one's identity is constant. Thomas suggested that compatibility genes could provide such an identifying mark – because they varied so much between individuals – and crucially, this seemed to fit with the Boyses' observations. So, as a team, they set out to test the hypothesis directly; by caging together different mice and simply observing who mated with whom – clearly, not an experiment that's ethically possible to do with humans.

The team's careful experiment confirmed their anecdotal observation – that when a mouse is presented with the choice of two potential mates, its preference is influenced by compatibility genes. But how? How did mice detect each other's compatibility genes? Smell was one possibility, and so Ted Boyse got in touch with a renowned expert in olfaction, Gary Beauchamp at the Monell Chemical Senses Center in Philadelphia, the largest research institute in the world specifically focused on understanding taste and smell.[13] They got to know each other over the coming decades, and when I spoke to Beauchamp in 2011, he said that he considered Ted Boyse nothing less than a genius. Boyse was always having original ideas, he recalled: beyond their experiments on smell, for example, Boyse also suggested using umbilical cord blood as a source of stem cells for transplantation, a brilliant idea which became widespread medical practice from the early 1990s.[14]

To study the mouse sense of smell, Boyse, Beauchamp and Thomas recruited a researcher from Japan, Kunio Yamazaki, to carry out a series of experiments using a Y-shaped tunnel (formally called a maze) equipped with a fan to blow different smells down each branch of the 'Y'. Mice placed at the bottom of the maze would run into one of the two branches of the 'Y' depending on the smell they preferred. To train mice to use the maze, the strong smells of juniper and cinnamon were blown down the branches, and mice were rewarded with a drink when they went down the Juniper-scented track. Next – again by offering appropriate rewards – mice could be successfully trained to smell other mice placed at the pronged end of the 'Y' who had either the same or different compatibility genes. This showed that mice were able to detect the type of compatibility genes another mouse had to make an appropriate choice and win a prize.

The team then found that they could repeat these kinds of experiments by replacing the actual mice being smelt at the prongs of the 'Y' with samples of their urine – again using fans to blow the scent down the tunnel. While this doesn't rule out other ways that mice sense compatibility genes, this showed that smelling urine is one way they can. Rats were also shown to be able to identify each other by smelling urine.[15] Thankfully, it's a skill lost in us.

Two big questions arose from this discovery: first, what do animals use their ability to sense each other's compatibility genes for; and second, is anything analogous true for humans? As for the first issue, we still don't know the answer – but there are several possibilities. One idea is that these genes could be used as a mark of kinship, employed by mice to avoid inbreeding or incest. Another possibility is that mice use these genes to find relatives for communal nesting – mothers may recognize their children this way, for example.[16] A third possibility is that mating preferences might specifically help keep immune-system genes diverse – since leaving different strains of mice to mate at will leads to offspring with more diverse compatibility genes than would be expected by chance.[17]

But what of the second question: how does this relate to humans? Can we also unconsciously assess the compatibility genes of potential partners? Are we secretly parading our genetic make-up to everyone around us by our smell, regardless of whether or not we choose to show off our status by flaunting wealth or good looks like peacocks?

Jon van Rood, one of the pioneers in HLA research, who we met in Chapter 3, among others, tried to test this in the 1980s, but his results were inconclusive because, as we've said, smell is inherently difficult to measure.[18] Then, in June 1994, Wedekind took up the challenge with a now infamous and provocative experiment.

He first established which types of compatibility genes a cohort of students had – forty-nine females and forty-four males.[19] The women – who happened to be mainly taking courses in biology or psychology – were then asked to take care of their sense of smell by using a nasal spray for fourteen days, and to sensitize their perception of smell by reading Patrick Süskind's fantasy novel *Perfume: The Story of a Murderer*. The men – mainly studying chemistry, physics or geography – were asked to wear a plain cotton T-shirt for two nights and refrain from anything that might affect their odour: sex, smoking, drinking alcohol, using deodorants or even entering a smelly room.

After these two nights, the men's worn T-shirts were placed in cardboard boxes with triangular holes. Then, alone in a room, each woman smelt six different T-shirts and ranked them on a scale of nought to ten (five meaning neutral and zero being unpleasant) against three criteria: intensity, pleasantness and sexiness.

But before the results had been analysed, there was already a problem. Journalists had picked up the scent of a good story. And some students who had received letters asking for their participation in the study thought that the research sounded dangerous and unethical. The second-largest newspaper in Switzerland at the time, *Berner Zeitung*, published an article quoting students protesting the project. One was reported to have said that the study was demeaning to women because this type of research implied that 'women's functions and abilities are reduced to reproduction'.[20] Another complained that the idea of anything influencing reproduction towards 'optimized' offspring is unsuitable as the subject of scientific research. Politicians panicked, and two phoned Wedekind.[21] One said that he had heard about Wedekind's 'Nazi research'. He said that the work must stop immediately – and that they would do everything in their power to have him removed from the University. Wedekind's superiors at the University took notice of the furore – but concluded that there was nothing wrong with the experiment.[22]

So, back in the lab, Wedekind and his co-workers analysed their data to compare preferences women had for T-shirts worn by men with similar or dissimilar compatibility genes – specifically HLA-A, -B and one of the class II HLA genes (chosen for being important in influencing transplantation success, hence tests for these genes were readily available). The outcome was that women ranked T-shirts to be more pleasant and sexier when worn by men with different compatibility genes from themselves. Women's rating for the *intensity* of smell didn't correlate with compatibility genes, confirming that it was *pleasantness* or *sexiness* that was important here. The experiment seemed to show that we unconsciously favour sexual partners who have different compatibility genes from ourselves.

And there was another dramatic result; woman taking a contraceptive pill didn't show the same preferences. In fact, their tastes were reversed, so that women taking the pill preferred men with similar compatibility genes to themselves. One way of interpreting this is that during pregnancy – to some extent mimicked by the effects of the contraceptive pill – selecting a sexual partner becomes unimportant, so preferences are altered and a pleasant smell might instead be associated with family members who have similar compatibility genes. Wedekind concluded that if mate preference was linked to our survival from disease then the 'negative consequences of disturbing this mechanism, by the use of perfumes and deodorants or by the use of the contraceptive pill during mate choice, need to be known by users'.

He sent his paper describing his research to the top scientific journals but ran into trouble again. One reviewer for *Nature* said that his method was simply not rigorous.[23] Papers in *Nature* usually report scientific methods as dispassionate protocols – with details about the dose of drug and the numbers of cells tested – not a method which stated that the subjects were first given a book to read. Wedekind's approach had the effect of seeming to dramatize his research – something every scientist is taught to avoid. Surely the results can't rely upon women reading a particular book, the *Nature* reviewer queried. Would results change if they were given a different book to read? The reviewers also questioned the effect of the nasal spray and the degree of acquaintance between people in the study. A more bizarre complaint was the suggestion that students might not be representative of humanity at large.[24]

Editors at another top journal, *Science*, didn't even consider the paper worthy enough for full peer review, and Wedekind finally had the study published in the UK's *Proceedings of the Royal Society*, a respectable journal to publish in but not in the premier league. A leading evolutionary theorist at Oxford University, Bill Hamilton, had suggested to Wedekind that he publish there after discussing the findings with him at a conference. In a letter to Wedekind, Hamilton said that sample sizes would ideally be larger but that, nevertheless, 'it is all fascinating and more needs to be done'.[25] Hamilton also said that a 'field for speculation here is that the pill may have a slow adverse effect on marital relations in the modern world . . . I seem to have seen effects that might be of this kind both in my own experience of relations with women and in that of close friends.'[26] Publication of these data – perhaps especially that the pill could influence a woman's sexual preference – was clearly going to cause a riot.

The study was indeed widely covered by the mainstream media as well as general science magazines[27] – but many scientists remained sceptical of the experiment. Talking to me in 2011, Wedekind thinks that this was because he and his co-authors worked outside the established community of researchers in immunology or HLA genetics.[28] That may be part of the problem, but to my mind the root of the cautious reception is the fact that the level of proof needed to persuade scientists of anything is roughly proportional to how important it is. If something doesn't have any consequence, then nobody will fuss over the details, but Wedekind's conclusions suggested a new aspect of human biology that was of huge public interest and of direct relevance to several multi-billion dollar industries from perfumeries to soap manufacturers. As the magician James Randi has said: if you claim to have a goat in your back yard, people might take your word for it, but if you say you have a unicorn, you can expect closer scrutiny.[29]

One spat was actually published, something that's uncommon, because most disagreements between scientists remain verbal – in arguments at scientific meetings. In this published disagreement, scientists criticized the statistical methods Wedekind had used to analyse

his data.[30] Wedekind responded by sending them the raw data to analyse themselves.[31] They then agreed that the conclusions remained the
same even when they analysed the data their own way; but the recon-
ciliation remains unpublished, and only the disagreement stays in
public view.[32] In any case, there was a far bigger problem than this for
Wedekind's experiment.

Statistical analysis shows whether or not something is likely to have
happened by chance, but it gives no indication to how important the
result is. Irrespective of the details about how statistical analysis
should be done – and whether or not some aspects of Wedekind's
method could have been improved, such as giving women a particular
book to read and so on – irrespective of all those concerns, even if the
results are taken at face value, their importance remains unclear;
because a score for the sexiness of smell is inherently difficult to
interpret.

The details of Wedekind's results are important here; the average
score each woman gave for the pleasantness of T-shirts worn by men
with dissimilar compatibility genes was just over five out of ten, whereas
for men with similar compatibility genes the average score was just
over four out of ten. Another way of analysing the same data is to say
that the average score each male received from women with dissimilar
compatibility genes was just under six out of ten, compared to nearly
five out of ten from women with similar genes. So the important point
is that – irrespective of whether or not the methods can be improved –
nobody knows whether or not a difference of a single point on a scale
of one to ten for the sexiness of a smell would actually influence a
person's behaviour. The evolutionary biologist Bill Hamilton got it
absolutely right when he concluded that it's all fascinating, but that
more needs to be done.

Now the *really* big problem is that subsequent research hasn't
exactly clarified the situation – in fact, more research has only added
numerous complications. Some studies have simply failed to detect
the effect that Wedekind found. One experiment very similar to Wedekind's, performed in 2008, showed that women's preferred smells
could indeed change when using the contraceptive pill, but that, in
general, dissimilarity in compatibility genes didn't correlate with
women's preferences.[33] Several differences in this later study, compared

to Wedekind's, could account for the change in result. For example, in this 2008 study, T-shirts were stored in a freezer before being smelt, whereas Wedekind had his T-shirts smelt quickly after being worn. So if the compatibility gene-related smell is lost over time or upon freezing, this additional step would have a big effect. Also, in the more recent experiment, women first smelt all the T-shirts before scoring each one separately whereas in Wedekind's experiment, women scored each T-shirt on first encounter. Nobody knows if this could subtly influence the outcome.

The 2008 study did, however, reveal a small increase in desire for men with similar compatibility genes for women taking the contraceptive pill – in agreement with Wedekind's results. Even so, conclusions about the use of the pill remain debatable. One issue that is hard to address, for example, is that correlation with women using the pill doesn't actually show that the pill directly changes women's preferences – it could also relate to other factors linked with using the pill such as one's relationship status or lifestyle.

Another experiment – this time by a team at the University of Chicago in Illinois in 2002 – came to the startling conclusion that a women's own compatibility genes influenced her preferences differently, according to which genes she had inherited from Mum or Dad.[34] The method for this experiment was familiar – T-shirts were worn by men for two days and then scored by women. The difference this time was the pleasantness of each T-shirt smell was compared with the compatibility genes of the women assessors *and their parents*. But another difference, compared to earlier studies, was that, in this study, the women were all from a particular religious community, the Hutterites, a tight-knit North American population with European ancestry who refrain from using oral contraceptives and have a relatively limited range in compatibility genes. The Hutterite women rated T-shirts worn by males from outside this community.

One conclusion from this study was that there wasn't any male smell that all or even most women liked or disliked; preferences varied. This is one reason why students and politicians needn't have panicked when they first heard about Wedekind's plans, because these studies show that diversity is what's important; there's no superior smell – everyone's gets preferred by someone. But the unexpected discovery from the study with Hutterite women was that they preferred the smell from men who had similar compatibility genes to their father. Preferences didn't correlate with her mother's genes – women liked men who smelt like Dad.

One eminent scientist commented that, with this discovery, the influence compatibility genes have on behaviours rivals their importance in immunity.[35] Yet these results seem to be the complete opposite result to Wedekind's earlier experiment, which found that women preferred *dissimilar* genes to their own. Just like others had done to him all those years before, Wedekind published a note complaining about the way that the statistical analysis was done in the study of Hutterite women – and the Chicago team simply replied to say that their analysis was appropriate.

In truth, these different results do not necessarily mean that one of the teams got it wrong. Behaviours influenced by compatibility genes may have several different roles – avoiding inbreeding, identifying close family to be cared for and maintaining diversity in the immune system. So whether or not a smell is regarded as pleasant, attractive or sexy may well depend on the environment and the atmosphere of the experiment, the way the question is asked and the culture of the people involved – all aspects that are very difficult to take account of. It seems feasible that in one type of situation women prefer the smell of T-shirts from men with related genes, while in another circumstance those worn by men with *different* genes smell sexier. We all know that feeling sexy is very much mood-orientated – so these studies may have arrived at different conclusions if they differed in subtle ways that affected how smells were perceived.

Given such difficulties, perhaps working out how we smell each other's compatibility genes would shed light on the situation; and *how* something works is usually easier for scientists to tackle – compared to *why*. One possibility is that HLA proteins (or peptides presented in their groove) are smelt directly. In mouse urine, fragments of these proteins have been found, and sensory neurons in the mouse nose have receptors that could mimic the receptors on immune cells that detect HLA proteins.[36] In humans, HLA proteins are found in blood. But they are not volatile (not easily changed to a vapour), so it's not obvious how they could be detected as an odour. An alternative

WBC/o

possibility is that compatibility genes may be sensed indirectly. Many scientists – including Wedekind – consider it likely that something volatile correlates with the versions of compatibility genes a person has inherited – and that's what can be directly smelt.

Most of the research to work out precisely how odour relates to compatibility genes has been in mice – because the use of inbred strains allows comparisons between mice with specific differences in their compatibility genes.[37] Two different types of experiments have been done: one approach is to capture the volatile chemicals emitted from mouse urine and analyse them to see if anything correlates with compatibility genes. The other idea has been to isolate the components of mouse urine and use them separately in two prongs of a Y-shaped maze to test which enable mice to still be able to distinguish compatibility genes. Despite all the effort – in both directions – a simple answer hasn't emerged. Huge effort by scientists is common; breakthroughs are rare.

There have been results that show some small volatile chemicals in mouse urine can correlate with compatibility, but there are inconsistencies between reports from different research teams. The problem is that the number of chemicals in mouse urine is vast. Even if the make-up of urine varies with mouse compatibility genes, it also differs according to the state of health of the animal, its age, body weight, food and water intake, urination frequency and so on. So for now, while there is considerable evidence that mice can detect each other's compatibility genes by smell, there's still no consensus about how they do it. Beauchamp at the Monell Chemical Senses Center concedes that it 'has been one of the great disappointments of my life – not knowing how it works'.[38]

However, this is not only a story of mice and men. Further down the animal kingdom, stickleback fish also use odours to choose a mate. Experiments analogous to the Y-shaped maze have been performed for fish – by taking water from tanks containing individual males and pumping it along different tracks that females could then choose between. This revealed that a sexy smell for stickleback fish is again influenced by compatibility genes – but there's a fascinating twist.[39]

Humans (and mice) have a fixed number of compatibility genes. It was our variability in these genes that was considered in Wedekind's T-shirt experiment and the like. But stickleback fish each have a different *number* of these genes. They can have between two and eight versions of one particular compatibility gene, which has been studied in detail. And instead of their preferred smell correlating to whether or not a potential mate had similar or dissimilar genes, the important factor is the *number* of these genes each individual fish has.

This behaviour is very likely aimed at achieving an optimal inheritance of immune-system genes, but it isn't as simple as, say, all fish prefer partners with high numbers of compatibility genes. There's a balance that determines how many of these genes is optimal for an immune system – something we discussed for humans in Chapter 5 to answer why we don't have, say, hundreds of HLA genes. Recall that having a larger number of different HLA proteins might be useful for being able to detect a greater number of foreign things in the body, but having too many makes it harder to ensure that there is not an inadvertent reaction to the body's own cells and tissues. A balanced immune system is best and – consistent with this idea – female sticklebacks with an already large number of compatibility genes were less keen on the smell from males who also had many genes; and those with few compatibility genes themselves were keen on the scent of males with more.[40]

In fact, six ends up being the number of these particular compatibility genes that stickleback fish inherit most often – though many have more or less than this. For this variability to exist, individual fish should be susceptible and resistant to different diseases according to the numbers of genes they have. That is, fish with few genes should be better at avoiding some diseases and those with many genes better at fighting others – in the same way that the sickle cell anaemia gene is kept in the population for its benefit against malaria even though it has the cost of potentially causing sickle cell anaemia (discussed in Chapter 5). There is evidence that this is the case: fish with few compatibility genes are more susceptible to certain parasites.[41] It is possible these same fish would be more resistant to other illnesses, but it has to be said that genetic factors influencing the course of disease in fish have been far less studied than, for example, the genes that affect HIV in humans. For mice and stickleback fish, compatibility genes play a role in selecting mates, in different ways for the different species.

For humans, it's commonly thought that our sense of smell is relatively feeble in comparison to many animals'.[42] In fact, it's debatable as to how feeble our sense of smell really is, but, more importantly, the way we choose a partner is driven by social conventions and culture to an extent that animals do not experience. So although all the research discussed so far could be taken to support the idea that compatibility genes can influence mate selection, none of these experiments so far address whether or not it is an *important* factor within the enormous complexity of how we choose our relationships.

One way to assess the overall impact of compatibility genes on human behaviour is to test whether or not married couples (or those in established relationships) have dissimilar or similar compatibility genes more frequently than would be expected by chance. Rose Payne – one of the early pioneers in HLA research, whom we met in Chapter 3 – studied this in 1983 and found that, in fact, couples were more likely to have similar compatibility genes.[43] This is the opposite of what would be expected following Wedekind's smelly T-shirt experiment, since his experiment indicated people would prefer partners with dissimilar genes. However, Payne's analysis involved many different ethnic groups and if people tended to partner with people of similar ethnicity – as was likely the case in the San Francisco area, where Payne's research was done – this alone would account for couples having *similar* HLA genes more frequently than expected by chance. One way to reconcile Payne's data with Wedekind's experiment is that our social and cultural conventions may swamp the influence of compatibility genes in how we choose partners.

In other studies, no correlation was found between compatibility genes and mate preferences. It could be that we should accept this at face value: that compatibility genes have little influence on who really settles down with whom. But scientists who advocate the importance of these genes in mate selection point out that HLA genes are just so diverse that the number of people studied may have been too small to detect their influence.[44]

One study in 1997, however, did find evidence to suggest that there may be a preference for couples to have dissimilar HLA types.[45] Interestingly, this research involved members of the religious Hutterite community, who are likely to be shielded from many social and cultural trends that are commonplace elsewhere – which could be an important factor in why an effect of compatibility genes was detected here. Also, this group has a limited range of compatibility genes, making their influence easier to pick out.

All in all, it is clear that compatibility genes influence mate selection in some animals. There is evidence – contentious evidence – that this can also happen in humans. But it is not yet clear how strongly this influences us: some scientists will argue very little; others argue forcefully for its importance. The biggest problem is that the way that compatibility genes are linked to smell – either in animals or humans – remains to be understood. To me, and many other scientists, molecular details in how this works – to understand how animals or humans 'smell' one another – are needed before we can clearly establish how big an influence compatibility genes are. But Beauchamp – who helped set up the early Y-shaped maze experiments – argues that this criticism isn't entirely fair: we know there's a specific odour of coffee even though we don't know exactly how it works.[46]

Even if compatibility genes are just one of many factors that influence our relationships, the implications are profound for understanding human biology. It's even possible that the compatibility gene system first evolved to allow individuals to distinguish kin from others and then later these genes were hijacked by the immune system to be used in the search for disease. Fundamentally, this research area expands how the human body can discriminate self from non-self – from the way Burnet first presented it in 1949 to an extent he never dreamed of. Compatibility genes might be used to distinguish self and non-self at a whole other level, influencing how we unconsciously sense family members, strangers or lovers.

More research is sorely needed. Yet this is just *one* hint that compatibility genes reach into human biology far more deeply than first thought. Next: your brain.

9

Connections with the Mind

Pink Floyd's rock album *The Wall* tells the metaphorical story of a wall we build around ourselves so that we don't expose our true passions. When society puts pressure on girls not to take an interest in science, it adds another brick in that wall. Neuroscientist Carla Shatz is acutely aware that this needs to change and she has led by example.

Shatz was the first female to get a PhD in neurobiology from Harvard and then the first female basic scientist to win a tenured position at Stanford Medical School – after being hired initially through an affirmative action policy to attract more women.[1] She achieved a similar feat yet again when she became the first woman to head Harvard's Department of Neurobiology. She loved Stanford and eventually moved back there but says of her Harvard job: 'I couldn't turn it down because I felt I was on a mission to represent women at the highest levels.'[2] Many scientists champion a cause beyond their own research, because it takes a similar strength of character to drive change in social attitudes as it does to cut a new path in scientific knowledge – both require a healthy disregard for the status quo to break down its walls.

From her position of authority, Shatz has worked hard to help others attain a good work–life balance. Not one size fits all, she says: some people need access to good childcare while some need help in getting employment for their partner.[3] She says that she knows all too well that juggling career and family is extremely challenging.[4] Yet her challenge turned out to be in *not* having a family. She had always assumed that she'd have children at some point but, with her career going so well, she ended up waiting too long.[5]

Having broken the glass ceiling in her career, Shatz smashed through another invisible barrier: the prevailing scientific doctrine. At the time, proteins encoded by compatibility genes were well established as being critical in the immune system, but they were thought to have nothing to do with neurons. Through a series of experiments carried out during the late 1990s, Shatz and her team discovered these genes do, in fact, work in the brain. The immediate implication was that that the wiring of our brains involves key proteins from our immune system – and, once again, our compatibility genes appeared more powerful than we once imagined.

Basic processes such as how cells get their energy are pretty similar in all kinds of different cell types, so it is to be expected that many genes and proteins will be active in both neurons and immune cells. But compatibility genes – and the proteins they encode for – weren't considered to participate in anything that cells do generally. They were considered to be especially adapted for a job in the immune system, so there was no reason to think they would be important in the brain. In fact, the textbook view of the time was that the brain was one of the privileged organs that are protected from immune reactions. So there was actually some reason to think that it was important that these proteins *not* be present in the brain.[6] The thinking behind this was that the brain is such an essential organ that it would be too risky to have immune cells patrolling as usual. Damage to the brain that might be caused by an immune reaction – and the inevitable destruction of diseased tissue – is likely to be so devastating that the possibility is best avoided. In support of this idea, entry of immune cells into the brain is tightly regulated by the so-called blood–brain barrier. However, we now know that an immune response can occur in some situations – and a common view today is that the brain is protected from immune responses to some extent, but not entirely.[7] In any case, Shatz's work wasn't revelatory for merely finding immune-system proteins in the brain – her research also indicated that these proteins were being used there for something that had nothing to do with fighting infection.

Shatz didn't arrive at this point by setting out to study the immune system or compatibility genes. She wanted to understand how images received by the eye are interpreted by the brain. A neuroscientist by training, she worked for her doctorate from 1971 to 1976 at Harvard University under the guidance of Canadian-born David Hubel and Swede

Tortsen Wiesel, who were at the time carrying out pioneering research which would later, in 1981, win them the Nobel Prize in Physiology or Medicine. Shatz joined their team, having been inspired by lectures she went to as an undergraduate student on the 'Chemistry of Vision' given by George Wald, famous for his research on understanding the retina (which won him a Nobel Prize in 1967). Shatz was fascinated by the question of 'how we see'. It combined her love of art and science.[8]

Shatz's PhD supervisors – Hubel and Wiesel – worked together for twenty-five years, from 1958 to 1983, to understand how our brain interprets what our eye 'sees'. In the human brain, there are about 20 billion individual cells or neurons making a quadrillion – that is 1,000,000,000,000,000 – connections, or synapses, between each other.[9] It is widely believed that the way in which contacts between neurons are configured underlies all emotion, thought and memory – somewhat similar to how the configuration of an electronic circuit determines what it does.

There was one crucial technical advance that allowed Hubel and Wiesel to probe which brain neurons fired when animals – usually cats – were shown different shapes projected onto a screen.[10] Hubel – a technical whizz – had crafted a small wire, or electrode, fine enough so that it could be used to detect the activity of a single neuron. The electrode could be hooked up to an instrument that recorded – or made a sound – when one individual neuron was activated.

With this technical advance, they uncovered a spectacular array of information about how vision works. The first striking observation they made was when Hubel noticed that neurons in the brain wouldn't do anything when he turned the lights on and off – but they would fire up when he waved his hand.[11] This opened the door to the complexity of how animals 'see'. Through a series of carefully planned experiments, the duo found, for example, that a particular neuron would react when the animal was shown a line of light orientated in a specific direction. That is, one particular brain cell would be activated when an animal was shown a line of light pointing to, say, the number two on a clock-face and not when it was rotated to point at numbers one or three. As well as this orientation-specific activation of neurons, they showed how movement of edges or borders was important in determining which brain cells fired. With this, Hubel and Wiesel could map out what they called the *functional architecture* of the visual cortex.

Before these discoveries, it had been assumed that what the eye saw was simply projected onto cells in the brain in some way – something like how an image is pixelated and displayed on a TV or computer screen. But Hubel and Wiesel found out that the visual field is processed and interpreted – so that, for example, a moving object is preferentially picked out from any non-changing background. It's what you experience when you catch something moving out of the corner of your eye – like a bird flying out from a tree that you were barely aware of. Their research begun to establish how the visual world is dissected and analysed by our brain.[12]

It's very rare that two scientists work so closely together over such a long period of time. Hubel said of their relationship that 'had it not been for Torsten's ability to keep his eye on the ball I might have squandered all my time playing with and designing equipment, rather than sticking to biology'. [13] A multitude of colourful characters have made seminal contributions to science, but Hubel and Wiesel only offer an apology 'for not having led more adventurous lives. Neither of us climbed Mount Everest, took part in the French Resistance, or sailed around the world.'[14] Science was their big adventure.

Francis Crick, co-discoverer of the double-helix structure of DNA, realized that Hubel and Wiesel had opened a window into the impossible jungle of the brain.[15] He had Hubel give a seminar to a small audience of ten leading molecular biologists at the Salk Institute, La Jolla, where Crick worked at the time. Scheduled for an hour but lasting for over three, the lecture ended with the select audience firing boundless questions at the speaker. The enthusiasm of such formidable scientists gave Hubel confidence and the feeling that his work was truly important or, in his own words, not so boring after all.[16] Crick – turned on by neuroscience – wanted to recruit Hubel to the Salk Institute. But Hubel wouldn't come without Wiesel, and Wiesel wouldn't come without another colleague who in turn wouldn't come without some of his co-workers. And negotiations evaporated. But Crick continued to meet Hubel fairly frequently and legend has it that Crick continued to edit his own final manuscript about the brain until the day he died in 2004.

Staying at Harvard, Hubel and Wiesel made many other important discoveries. They observed, for example, that different patches of cells towards the back of the brain responding to signals from the left or right eye. When they covered one eye, they found that a young animal's brain could restructure these bands of cells and devote more neurons to signals from the open eye. This showed that a basic wiring of the visual part of the brain is present at birth but, importantly, it is not fixed for ever. Rather, the organization of this part of the brain develops during a critical early period in life, in response to what the eyes see. This research established that the cellular structure of the brain *can change*.

It was this activity-dependent restructuring of the brain that Shatz wanted to study. She wanted to understand exactly how it occurred, to identify which genes and proteins were switched on to develop the brain in response to signals from the eye.

For Shatz, this was a way into exploring the broad issue of how our brains change through learning and experience; a step towards understanding how the construction of the brain results from an entanglement of nature (genes) and nurture (cues from what the eye sees). Shatz sees this issue as being the key to figuring out what the brain is all about – because it's this adaptability or plasticity that makes the brain so much more than just an ultra-powerful computer. In effect, by rearranging the connections between neurons, experience alters the hardware of a brain – something that doesn't happen in man-made electronic circuitry.[17]

Shatz decided that the best way to attack the problem was to use drugs to block neural activity during development of the visual part of a cat's brain – and determine which genes altered their activity as a result. This, in effect, gave her a list of genes activated when brain cells respond to cues from the retina. Unexpectedly, she found increased activity of compatibility genes correlated with neuronal activity, which indicated that these immune system genes could have a role in structuring this part of the brain.[18]

She submitted her discovery to be considered for publication in *Nature*. However, after a short time, an editor wrote back to her to say that he wouldn't be able to publish the study or even send it out for in-depth peer review. He had bounced the paper off two experts in immunology and both had said there must be something wrong with the work because everybody already knows that neurons don't use these genes; they're only important in the immune system.[19] This reaction from *Nature* made her realise that she was pitching a story that went against a powerfully guarded dogma – and she would need more evidence to convince people.

Pursuing the research in cats was difficult because feline genes had been relatively little studied. So Shatz switched to studying mice – where defined genetic variants are obtained easily. She realized that she could use mice which had already been bred to lack proteins encoded by compatibility genes; such mice had been used to establish the importance of these proteins for survival against infections. Shatz could examine what these mutations did to the structure of the mouse brain, something that nobody had ever thought to look at before, despite having the mice available for years.

Although these mice looked normal on the outside, upon dissection Shatz found abnormalities in the way the visual part of the brain was organized.[20] She saw a higher number of connections between neurons than found in normal mice. Too many neuronal connections suggested that MHC proteins were important in pruning synapses that weren't appropriate when this part of the brain developed. Her team also looked at another mutant mouse, which this time lacked a protein known to be important in white blood cells. She found the same alteration in brain structure, implying that other proteins used by immune cells are also important in the brain.

Her background – working with Hubel and Wiesel – led Shatz to focus on the visual part of the brain; but a question arising from her initial findings was whether or not it was *only* the visual part of the brain that gets affected in this way. To answer this, her team decided to look somewhere else in the brain: the hippocampus, the place where connections between neurons strengthen or weaken as memories form. In the mice that were defective in producing MHC proteins, stimulation of neurons in the hippocampus resulted in abnormally strong signals. This suggested that compatibility genes could have a role outside the visual part of the brain, affecting the area important for consolidating long-term memories.

Shatz concluded that neuronal connections in parts of the brain – even in the hippocampus – could be influenced by proteins previously thought to work in the immune system. And the reaction from other scientists? Most were cautious and sceptical, reminiscent of the reaction to Wedekind's smelly T-shirt experiment a few years earlier. Suggesting that MHC proteins are important in structuring the brain felt like someone claiming they have a unicorn in their garden – it warranted close scrutiny.

It's not that anybody would consider Shatz's data as being deliberately falsified (fraud actually happens rarely in science, and only about 300 papers are formally retracted from around 1.4 million published annually),[21] but rather that scientists know all too well that not everything that gets published turns out to be right – for any number of reasons. An experimenter might have been deceived by their own bias; reagents or chemicals might not have worked exactly as thought; experiments might have had inadequate controls; or, worst of all, scientists might have thought up some excuse to leave out part of the data that didn't fit their story – ignoring the fact that at a high dose, for example, a particular drug did something that didn't fit their hypothesis, and only publishing what happened when it was used at a low dose. It's not always straightforward to tell right from wrong in published papers because scientists present their work as a 'story' based on a long series of complex experiments, and anything that doesn't fit their 'narrative' often gets left out.

For Shatz's work, the main source of contention was the lack of anyone having a detailed understanding about *how* the MHC proteins could influence organization of neuronal synapses in the brain. For any phenomenon that strays from what's expected, biologists like a good explanation of how it works before taking the new idea as fact; as the mantra goes: show me how it works before I believe it's true. Although sceptical, most scientists were intrigued, and if she *was* right then a burning issue was whether or not this reflected a trivial recycling of molecules to be used for a different task or whether, instead, this cracked open a fundamental link between our nervous and immune systems.

Given that compatibility genes – and the proteins they encode – vary so much, it might seem unlikely for the brain to co-opt such a complex system unless their variability was somehow important for their role in the brain. But this argument is flawed. Because it requires that we – and other living things – have evolved to end up working in an efficient or sensible way. In fact, there are many examples in nature where things work fine without being slick like an iPad. The way that we have been formed – through a process of evolution – means that everything must be built upon what went before, not constructed elegantly from scratch.

Take, for example, the path of a particular thin tube in men called the *vas deferens*, which transports sperm from the testicles to the urethra (it's the connection that's severed in a vasectomy). Instead of this tube taking a straight path, it follows a route far longer than it needs to by looping over another bit of tubing in the area, the ureter. There doesn't seem to be any reason why it couldn't follow a direct path; it just happened to evolve to go the long way round. This has been explained by suggesting that the position of the testicles changed as we evolved from our ancestors and as that move occurred, the *vas deferens* tube got caught *over* the ureter rather than going *under* it. So, things don't evolve to a perfect design, and that's why it can't be taken for granted that the brain uses the same molecules as the immune system for any fundamental reason; it may have just happened to evolve that way. To claim that the connection between our immune and nervous systems is intimate – and not just a chance recycling of parts – there needs to be specific evidence.

We've discussed in detail how compatibility genes are linked to susceptibility or resistance to various types of infectious diseases, but also our variation in these genes has been linked to many neurological disorders, such as schizophrenia or bipolar disorder.[22] This is consistent with an intimate connection between compatibility genes and our nervous system. But researchers studying schizophrenia, and other neurological diseases, differ in their view of how important these genes are. Although many tens of studies link compatibility genes to schizophrenia, dispute remains because each comes to a different conclusion about which versions of these genes are risk factors for the illness.[23] This might reflect different diagnostic criteria used in studies: mental illnesses are notoriously difficult to categorize, and it is possible that different compatibility genes are important in particular versions of these multi-faceted diseases. There are at least three ways in which compatibility genes could, in principle, influence neurological illnesses.

An infection may underlie some mental illnesses; and then one way in which compatibility genes would be linked to neurological diseases is through their normal role in immune defence. In this scenario, the situation is identical to how these genes affect our susceptibility or resistance to other infectious diseases, such as AIDS. A second possibility is typified by the rare sleeping disorder narcolepsy, which has one of the strongest links of any disease to our HLA genes. About 1 in 2,000 people are affected so that their brain is unable to regulate the normal cycle of being awake and asleep.[24] Sufferers can fall asleep at inappropriate times during the day and sleep poorly at night. The vast majority of people with narcolepsy have particular versions of class II compatibility genes.[25] These versions of compatibility genes are found in almost all people with narcolepsy, but they are also common in those without the disease – so they are *not sufficient* to cause the illness and instead play some role in how it starts.

For some sufferers, there is evidence that narcolepsy is an autoimmune disease. That is, it arises because the immune system mistakenly attacks the body's own healthy tissue. Symptoms could be caused by an immune reaction against the neurons that are important for regulating sleep and wakefulness. In support of this, a protein made by neurons triggers an immune reaction in narcolepsy patients.[26] So HLA proteins could influence our susceptibility to narcolepsy according to the extent that they aid an immune attack on healthy neurons.

The third way in which these proteins could influence neurological disorders directly relates to Shatz's discovery: that these proteins can influence the way in which neuronal connections or synapses are configured in the brain. One possibility of how this might relate to disease stems from the fact that, during any kind of immune reaction in the body, immune cells secrete proteins – called cytokines. Cytokines do many things to help the immune reaction, one of which is to increase the production of MHC proteins. So if cytokines were secreted from immune cells at a time when these MHC proteins are important in sculpting the developing brain, it is feasible that the change in their production could lead to abnormalities in the structure of the brain.[27] But this is only an idea – nothing more than a feasible way in which compatibility genes link with neurological illness. Sadly, the causes of most mental illnesses remain baffling.

Aside from disease, Shatz's discovery also begs the question of whether or not compatibility genes affect normal brain functions – perhaps in some way that's more subtle than influencing the course of illness. Since her observations indicated that MHC proteins were important in how the brain changed in response to external stimuli – both in the visual cortex and then in the hippocampus – Shatz and her team decided to next investigate, in 2008, whether or not MHC proteins affect learning, a process that must involve changes to the brain.

It's exceptionally difficult – perhaps impossible – to test whether or not immune system genes influence how well humans learn, but Shatz could more easily explore the idea in mice. First, Shatz clarified which types of compatibility genes were being used in the mouse brain. The genes that vary enormously among us – HLA-A, -B, -C and so on – are called *classical* compatibility genes. But there are also a number of other genes – in humans and animals alike – that encode similarly shaped proteins which don't vary much between us. These are named the *non-classical* compatibility genes. Shatz's earlier work didn't distinguish between these different types of compatibility genes, but for their investigation into learning her team focused on the genes in mice that are equivalent to our HLA-A and -B genes – the classical compatibility genes that vary hugely in individual mice or people.

Mice genetically altered to lack these variable genes did indeed have defects in the cerebellum at the base of the brain. Specifically, synapses were not weakened in the right way, reminiscent of what she had discovered in other parts of the brain. The cerebellum is important for motor learning – how we learn skills by practising like riding a bike. Although we have little idea about how it works in any detail, it's generally accepted that motor learning will somehow require a reconfiguration of the connections between neurons – some being strengthened while others weaken. So if compatibility genes can influence which synapses weaken in the cerebellum, Shatz reasoned, could they affect the ability of mice to actually learn a skill?

To test this directly, Shatz's team used a simple apparatus called a Rotarod – a horizontal cylinder that rotates, on which mice can learn to balance so that they don't fall off. It's not harmful for the mice because the bar isn't so high that it hurts when they fall. But timing how long an individual mouse can stay balanced on the bar is a way of measuring their ability. After some practice, normal mice were able to stay on the rotating rod for around a minute, but mice lacking the equivalent genes to our HLA-A and –B genes could learn to balance for nearly double that time.[28] A lack of these genes isn't something that occurs naturally, but, by deliberately testing what does happen if they are missing, this experiment revealed that compatibility genes can influence the ability of mice to learn.

Mice lacking these genes also remembered their skill for much longer because, after a four-month break from practising, they were still much better at balancing on the rod. How would our hero from Chapter 1, Peter Medawar, have reacted if a know-it-all alien had visited and whispered: Peter, the genes you're studying – those that control the transplantation reaction – also work to fight infections, help organize the brain and influence learning? Still, stunning as these results are, there are at least two caveats – both of which Shatz acknowledges herself. First, it remains unknown whether or not humans (not just mice) use MHC proteins in this way in the brain; the problem is that it's very hard to think up an ethically sound experiment to test these ideas on people. Second, Shatz's experiments only show that the brain is affected in mice whose compatibility genes are *completely* incapacitated – an artificial situation just to test what happens if these proteins are removed. This doesn't really tell us whether or not the brain could be influenced by the natural diversity in these genes. If there is an effect caused by differences in these genes it is surely going to be subtle, compared to when these genes are incapacitated.

Our understanding of compatibility genes in the brain has simply not yet benefited from the decades it took for everyone to agree, for example, the importance of Medawar and Burnet's work. It is simply too soon for there to be unanimous agreement over the importance of Shatz's observations (or pretty much anybody else's discovery made within the last decade or so). Almost every statement in any scientific textbook is the outcome of many years' hard work and debate; and MHC proteins working in the brain is beyond current textbook-level science. While many scientists would argue that a popular-level book like this one should also stick to established decades-old ideas, my view is that nothing can be more exciting than what's happening at the edge of knowledge.

And most questions about the brain are at the edge of our knowledge, but the field is ripe for breakthroughs in the twenty-first century.

More than 32,000 people attended a neuroscience congress held in Washington, DC, in 2011, for example, while the same meeting forty years earlier attracted just over 1,000 people.[29] No other scientific discipline enjoys such stadium-sized lectures; Shatz says it feels like everyone's becoming a neuroscientist. When she first presented her data indicating that compatibility genes are active in the brain, in 1998, it was as a lone mention of the subject, but the neuroscience congress in 2011 was chock-full of presentations about how immune-system genes influence the brain and nervous system.[30] In fact, many components of our immune system are now known to influence our nervous system.

Receptors that immune cells use to detect bacteria, for example, can affect the extent of brain damage that occurs in a stroke.[31] This, with several related discoveries, has established that stroke and many other neurological problems can be triggered or exacerbated by immune responses. The medical implication is that targeting immune-system components might help. Drugs that block secretions from immune cells (cytokines), for example, could alleviate the symptoms caused by neuronal injury in stroke or brain trauma.[32] That Shatz helped establish connections between immune and nervous systems that soon might be medically useful must be gratifying, but when I put this to her in November 2011, she replied that, 'like all discoveries, first everyone says it's wrong, then everyone finds it out for themselves, and eventually everybody forgets that you made the discovery in the first place'.[33]

With hindsight, it maybe shouldn't have been so surprising that molecules are shared between our immune and nervous systems. These systems must be intimately connected; we've all experienced feeling sad or sleepy when ill. Indeed, immune responses are connected to all kinds of physiological processes.[34] In times of stress, for example, steroid hormones are released to alter energy use around the body and increase blood-sugar levels. These same hormones also dampen immune responses. They switch off excessive inflammation, which can damage tissues unnecessarily – this underlies the use of steroid hormones in preventer inhalers for asthma, to dampen immune responses in airways. A release of adrenaline triggered after an acute injury has the opposite effect; it stimulates or primes immune cells for action.

The interaction between our nervous and immune systems goes in both directions, as secretions from immune cells also affect the brain and central nervous system (and are the likely cause of us feeling sad and sleepy when ill). In fact, there is a vast web of neuro-immune circuitry that is critical to our well-being. Exercise, for example, affects the levels of various hormones and other proteins that circulate through blood, including adrenaline and cortisol levels, which in turn influence immune responses.[35] Regular exercise can have an anti-inflammatory effect, for example, which can protect against diseases in which a chronic immune response is part of the problem – such as in type 2 diabetes.

More research in this area is important but in deciding what next to do – where to target funding – it's useful to remember that Shatz's discovery came from exploration into how vision works, not a specific attempt to study the intersection between the immune and nervous systems, nor a direct effort to tackle any specific disease. Sparks might emerge from fostering greater interaction between scientists working in silos for understanding either immune cells or neurons. Much can be learned by thinking about the differences and similarities between these two types of cell.

In 1994, immunologists Bill Paul and Bob Seder at the National Institute of Health in Bethesda wrote a speculative but hugely influential article suggesting that neurons and immune cells have some similarity in how they work.[36] They reached this view because of an experiment that others performed in 1988 which showed that immune cells could secrete molecules in a specific direction, something that neurons had long been known to do.[37] The importance of this was in showing that immune cells and neurons can affect another cell in contact, rather than all the cells in the vicinity. Soon after Paul and Seder's article was published, Abraham 'Avi' Kupfer, working alongside his wife Hannah at the National Jewish Medical and Research Centre in Denver, performed experiments which directly showed a striking similarity in the way in which immune cells and neurons work.[38]

Kupfer's discovery came through watching immune cells in action with a high-powered microscope. In 1995, he stood before an unsuspecting crowd of a few hundred immunologists gathered for one of the prestigious Keystone symposia – named after a US ski resort where the meetings are often held. He showed images of immune cells interacting with other cells which revealed that the contacts between them involved aggregates of proteins organized into bull's-eye patterns.[39] His images showed two cells in contact – like two balls squashed together – and across the flattened connection between the two cells a patch of one protein coloured red could be seen surrounded by a ring of another protein labelled green. Before that moment, nobody thought these proteins would arrange themselves into a pattern at the contact between cells – but it was reminiscent of the organization of molecules at neuronal synapses.

This led to the common use of the term 'immune synapse' to describe the contacts that immune cells make with other cells. Both types of synapse involve rings of proteins to promote adhesion between cells and patches of other proteins particular to the discussion between the cells. To the Keystone audience, Kupfer's pictures were instantly accessible, and the immediate implication was that our thoughts and the detection of a virus both work through a complex choreography of molecules at the contacts between cells. One immunologist in the audience, Anton van der Merwe from Oxford University, remembers the event well:

> I recall us looking at these beautiful images for the first time in stunned silence. Although his talk overshot the allotted time no one showed any sign of leaving. After he had finished there was prolonged applause followed by many questions. When the chairperson ended the question session many of us crowded around Avi to continue the discussion.[40]

Independently, Mike Dustin, then at Washington University School of Medicine, St Louis, and his collaborators were also imaging immune cells but with an interesting twist. Instead of imaging two cells interacting together, they replaced one of the cells with a surrogate membrane composed of the lipids or fat molecules from a real cell but laid out flat on a glass slide. As immune cells landed on this glass-slide-supported mimic of a cell surface, they could also see dramatic movements of proteins labelled with different-coloured dyes. This artificial system was easier to image because the microscope could rapidly capture pictures of the flat synapse laid out over the glass slide. Their approach revealed that the immune synapse is dynamic so that arrangements of proteins change when, for example, a T cell responds to the presence of non-self (peptide).[41]

My contribution to the story of compatibility genes comes here. While working with Jack Strominger at Harvard University, independently from Kupfer and Dustin, I also discovered a structured immune synapse – but this time, formed by human Natural Killer cells.[42] I vividly recall looking at a computer screen, which relayed what was being detected down the microscope, to see patterns of differently coloured proteins at the contact between cells. Unsure of my ability to make an important discovery, I had to ask my girlfriend at the time (now my wife), who isn't a biologist, to come into the lab and use the microscope herself – to be sure I wasn't doing anything wrong. My research showed that synapses were important for different types of immune cell – and showed that different organizations of the synapse can switch immune cells on or off. The new science opened up by my research – together with Kupfer and Dustin – is that changing arrangements of molecules control immune-cell interactions, turning them on and off when needed, analogous to what happens at neuronal synapses.

One important difference between neuronal and immune synapses is that nerve cells sustain connections for very long periods of time – often years – while immune cells are specialized in making relatively brief contacts with other cells. An immune cell must assess the state of health of another cell very quickly and move on. An immune cell can kill a single tumour cell or virus-infected cell as fast as in five to ten minutes before moving on to check the next cell.

As well as forming synapses, another thing that nerve cells specialize in is using long protrusions or axons to connect with other cells that are far away. The textbook view of immune cells is that they don't do this; axons are something special for neurons. But again, the textbooks probably don't have the whole story, and immune cells may actually physically connect with other cells over long distances – albeit in a more transient fashion. My research team and others have observed that long tubes made of cell membrane do readily form between immune cells and other cells.[43] I called these connections 'membrane nanotubes', and they could constitute a new mechanism for communication between cells that are far apart. A cost of having these connections is that viruses such as HIV may use these connections to efficiently spread between cells.[44] Dangerous proteins that can cause mad cow disease, called prions, can also move between cells along nanotubes.[45] But these nanotubes are hard to detect – because they are so thin – and it remains an open question as to when and where they occur in the body; this is at another edge of our knowledge.[46]

Whether or not this particular detail about immune cells turns out to be important, it is already clear that our immune and nervous systems intersect at many levels. They must work in unison – because many molecular components and cell structures are shared. And this is a theme that emerges from much contemporary research in human biology. As we seek to understand how the billion proteins in an average cell allow them to move, multiply, create a brain or defend us against viruses and bacteria, we are beginning to discover how so many aspects of our bodies are intimately connected. The Human Genome Project revealed that we each have around 25,000 genes, which was a far smaller number than most scientists had predicted before the project began. And now we see why: *because genes multi-task*, making it inevitable that disparate aspects of us are interconnected.

The link between our immune and nervous systems through our compatibility genes is especially intriguing, because these genes vary so much between us. We know that these differences matter in our immune system and there's the possibility that something of our brains could be affected as well. However, there's simply no escaping the fact that we haven't got this all worked out; knowledge always ends somewhere, and that's never satisfying. To know more, you have three options: 1. sit back and wait patiently; 2. put on a lab coat and try to dig deeper yourself; or 3. encourage children to wonder, and maybe they'll figure it out. Perhaps we should have known from the beginning that any chapter about the brain would have to end too soon; everyone knows that there are more questions than answers in brain science. As Hubel said,

We breathe, cough, sneeze, vomit, mate, swallow, and urinate; we add and subtract, speak, and even argue, write, sing, and compose quartets, poems, novels, and plays; we play baseball and musical instruments. We perceive and think. How could the organ responsible for doing all that not be complex?[47]

Little in human biology is as miraculous as the brain. But birth must at least come close. And guess what: our compatibility genes turn up there too.

10

Compatibility for Successful Pregnancy

The idea behind this chapter doesn't really need words that are poetic, personal, colourful or clever because it is explosive enough said plain and simple: our variable immune system genes influence whether or not pregnancy is successful. Couples having certain combinations of immune-system genes are more likely to miscarry or have other problems in pregnancy. This extends the reach of compatibility genes into a whole other realm of human biology and links two of the most powerful natural forces that control human existence – survival from disease and successful reproduction.

Pregnancy has long been recognized as a problem for the immune system. Peter Medawar is often credited with bringing the issue into focus in an influential article published in 1953.[1] From his experiments – and the theories of his contemporary Burnet – he knew that detection of non-self can trigger an immune reaction, and this is what causes transplant rejection. Medawar realized that a foetus has half its genes from its father – so why doesn't the mother's immune system attack the foetus for being different, just like in a transplant? Every baby in every mother's womb must survive *against* the normal rules for successful transplantation. And so – Medawar reasoned – pregnancy presents a paradox, because a mother must nourish, not reject, tissue that is genetically different from her own.

Medawar considered that the most likely solution to this paradox is an anatomical separation of the foetus from its mother, but he never made much headway into exploring any details.[2] He was right that there is no direct contact between an embryo and its mother: a baby develops within an amniotic sac, and its blood circulation is kept separate from the mother's. The place where genetically different cells derived from the foetus could meet the mother's immune system is in the placenta, the organ which grows for nine months to connect the developing baby and the mother through the umbilical cord. The placenta is where an immune reaction must be prevented – and where the answer to Medawar's paradox must lie.

The human placenta lies on one side of the mother's uterus (or womb) and its main job is to allow nutrients and gases to pass between the mother and baby. The structure of the placenta – and birth in general – varies a lot between animals. While this is a great source of wonder for anyone fascinated by the diversity of life on earth, these differences are a source of frustration for scientists trying to work out basic principles of pregnancy. This is one area of human biology for which studies in animals are of limited use.[3] But, unlike most other human organs, it's relatively easy to obtain a human placenta, and so we know a great deal about the cells that go to make the placenta and its overall anatomy.

In the human placenta, maternal blood flows over a tree of finger-like projections, or villi, made from cells derived from the foetus. These villi contain foetal blood – to collect gases and nutrients – and are coated on the outside with cells that are called *trophoblast* cells. These trophoblast cells are, in effect, foetal cells that are in direct contact with the mother. A second type of cell from the foetus also contacts the mother's tissue – they are called *extra-villous trophoblast* cells. These foetal cells directly invade the mother's uterus and affect the walls of her arteries to help make sure that there is blood flow sufficient enough for nutrients to be absorbed by the foetus.[4] Where these trophoblast and extra-villous trophoblast cells from the embryo contact the mother, two individuals are connected in the most intimate way possible.

From this, the answer to Medawar's paradox is reduced to understanding trophoblast cells. A solution to the problem would be if trophoblast cells come into contact with the mother's blood but not her immune cells. That is, if the mother's immune cells are prevented from entering the uterus during pregnancy, making the uterus a privileged site in the body like the eye and the testis – special places where immune responses are prevented from occurring. Rupert Billingham – from Medawar's holy trinity – was one prominent scientist who explored this idea during the 1960s. But he found out, as did others, that immune cells can reach the uterus during pregnancy and infections can be fought there.[5] This isn't the answer.

Part of the true solution to Medawar's paradox is that trophoblast cells derived from the foetus are different from almost all other types of cell in that they are not able to trigger a strong immune response. Specifically, trophoblast cells don't make the proteins HLA-A and HLA-B, while almost all other types of cell in the body do. Trophoblast cells still make the HLA-C protein,[6] but by lacking HLA-A or HLA-B, there's not much for the mother's T cells to look at on trophoblast cells. In this way, they can avoid switching on the mother's T cells.

The situation is reminiscent of how some viruses infect cells and interfere with HLA proteins so that T cells can't detect that anything's wrong. But when that happens, another arm of your immune system spots the problem. Recall how Natural Killer (NK) cells can be activated by detecting 'missing self'; a loss of HLA proteins at the surface of cells can itself be taken as a sign of trouble. So if trophoblast cells inherently lack HLA proteins to avoid an immune reaction from the mother's T cells, why wouldn't they instead activate the mother's NK cells?

One solution to this conundrum would be if a mother's NK cells don't enter her uterus during pregnancy, even if other immune cells do. And so this begs the question of which kinds of immune cells there are in the uterus. Three pioneering British women answered this question independently in the late 1980s. One was Ashley Moffett, working at the time with Malaysian-born Yung Wai (Charlie) Loke at the University of Cambridge.[7] Loke was already in his fifties while Moffett was not yet an established scientist, having focused her career instead on clinical medicine. Loke and Moffett's story – a long partnership which began with Moffett's observations about which type of immune cells are present in the uterus – leads us to the unexpected link between the immune system and pregnancy.

Born in 1934, Loke had taught medicine in Malaysia before being recruited to Cambridge in 1967, where he had earlier been a student and where he then stayed thirty-five years, until retiring in 2002. His reputation was established in 1986, by being the first to isolate trophoblast cells from a human placenta so that they could be studied in detail. Moffett says that Loke is just as happy 'in a sarong, a tweed jacket or his scarlet academic gown'.[8]

Loke had had a distant relationship with his parents and was looked after by nannies during his early childhood. From age thirteen, he went to boarding school in the UK. He had wanted to be a marine biologist but ended up in medicine because he was taught at boarding school that medicine – unlike marine biology – was a proper career. Also at boarding school, he was given his name – Charlie – because nobody could pronounce Yung Wai. He has always remained an outsider. Even though he spent so long in Cambridge, he would often feel excluded when a conversation centred on an aspect of society he didn't know much about, sometimes bringing on a deep loneliness in the company of friends and colleagues.[9]

Before being sent to boarding school in the UK, Loke and his family fled from Malaysia to Singapore when it was captured by the Japanese in 1941. He moved again and lived under Japanese occupation in Kuala Lumpur with scarce resources and a diet of brown rice.[10] Memories of people being moved against their will influenced him ever after. He would always refrain from joining organized sightseeing tours often arranged during a scientific congress because he didn't like the idea of being shepherded about in a large group against one's free will.[11] His passion for freedom included making sure that his thinking was never trapped in paradigm.[12]

In fact, Loke was about as free as any scientist could be. He came from an exceptionally wealthy family, his grandfather having founded the tin and rubber industries in Malaysia. So, if he didn't get a particular research project funded through the normal peer-review system, he could just fund the work himself.[13]

At the time they began to work together, Moffett had only recently returned to work after a five-year career break during which time she had three children.[14] She had first met Loke while she was an undergraduate student; Moffett being one of about twenty women studying medicine with nearly 250 men.[15] Moffett had trained as a neurologist but took a job as the pathologist in a Cambridge maternity hospital, simply because it was all that was available. Quickly, she realized that a maternity hospital is a hectic environment to work in: babies are born round the clock without any consideration for sociable working hours. Her duty was to diagnose problems in pregnancy from biopsies and medical notes, but when Moffett queried how the biopsies actually related to the underlying causes of problems in pregnancy, nobody seemed to know; nobody had time to think about it. Biopsies could provide tell-tale signatures of particular problems in pregnancy, but nobody knew what caused such characteristics.

Moffett was often half asleep – with babies on her mind at work and at home – but she wanted to understand what happens when pregnancies didn't work out, and pre-eclampsia was one problem she came across frequently. It is a condition caused by abnormalities in implantation, resulting in poor blood flow in the placenta and high blood pressure in the mother. Left unchecked, it can lead to eclampsia, with symptoms that include seizures and coma – and which can be fatal. Looking through the biopsies, Moffett couldn't help but wonder why some women have this problem and others don't. And it felt unfair to her that other medical problems were studied so much more intensely. She felt that there was a gravitas given to, say, research in cancer – even relatively rare cancers – that just didn't seem to apply to studying pre-eclampsia, even though it affects 6–8 per cent of pregnancies. Pre-eclampsia can often be resolved with speedy delivery of the baby by caesarean section or induction of birth, but occasionally an abortion is necessary. The intervention saves lives, but premature birth of babies can sometimes lead to other problems – and the root cause of the problem is left unchecked. Moffett felt that if pre-eclampsia was a male problem, it wouldn't have been so under-studied.[16]

Each time she brought her microscope into focus, she didn't just seek a diagnosis, she looked for clues as to what *caused* pre-eclampsia. One thing she noticed over the slides she examined was that immune cells in the uterus were often particularly speckled or granular. Other scientists had already found immune cells present where foetal trophoblast cells invade a mother's uterus, but their identity was unclear. Moffett had read that an unusually speckled appearance was characteristic of NK cells – recall that this was the trait used to identify human NK cells in the first place. In 1987, she decided to go and see

Loke, the renowned local expert in the placenta – to tell him that she had discovered a lot of NK cells present in the uterus during pregnancy. She expected the old master to be flabbergasted – but his response was simply: what are NK cells?[17]

Loke wasn't ignorant. Rather it was a time when NK cells were relatively little known. Kärre's idea for the way in which NK cells detect diseased cells – the 'missing self' hypothesis – was only beginning to be debated. Loke got up to speed on NK cells and he invited Moffett to leave her hospital work and take up research full time in his laboratory. He mentioned that, if she really proved that NK cells are abundant in the uterus, she would probably never return to patient care. Moffett agreed to take a short sabbatical in 1987 and Loke's prediction proved right; she never did return to clinical medicine.

In Loke's lab, Moffett examined the uterine immune cells by systematically comparing stains for different kinds of cell and confirmed that a huge fraction of them were NK cells. They published their observations in a relatively obscure specialist journal.[18] Neither Loke nor Moffett was ambitious in a career-focused way and they never thought it important to seek a higher-profile place to publish.[19] The two others who discovered the presence of NK cells in the mother's uterus around the same time as Moffett were Judith Bulmer at Newcastle University and Phyllis Starkey at the University of Oxford.[20] Bulmer works as a clinical consultant for placental pathology, while Starkey left science to pursue a career in politics, becoming a Labour Member of Parliament in 1997 – it gave her 'a chance to change people's lives for the better'.[21] It probably helped her in politics that she had training in science like it helps in science to be good at politics.

It isn't just coincidence that much of the research described earlier in this book was male-dominated, while here women take the lead. In the six decades over which this story has unravelled, the role of women in science has improved considerably – a trend likely to continue as the stereotype of the male scientist becomes outdated and ignored. All three women, however, published their discovery about the placenta in specialist journals which weren't read by the mainstream NK-cell research community. The first time NK-cell researchers heard of this discovery was when Moffett presented her data in a poster at the NK-cell congress held in St Petersburg, Florida, in 1992. Discussion at that meeting centred on how NK cells detect diseased cells – and Kärre's idea of NK cells looking for 'missing self' was beginning to be accepted. All research on human NK cells at that time was done using cells isolated from blood. Moffett's suggestion that NK cells were also abundant in the uterus was met with bemusement. At that time, these meetings were male-dominated, and by far the most common question asked about her discovery was simply: 'What is a uterus?'[22]

Nowadays, the presence of so many NK cells is known to be a characteristic change to the uterus caused by the hormone progester-one. NK cells accumulate as part of the monthly cyclical changes that occur in the uterus and they die off a couple of days before menstru-ation, or stay if pregnancy occurs. Rather than 'What is a uterus?', the important question to be asked is 'What are all these NK cells doing there?' NK cells specialize in detecting a loss of compatibility protein from cells, which is exactly the case for trophoblast cells – so what stops these NK cells from attacking these cells in the placenta?

There's one very special thing about trophoblast cells which looks to be important for resolving this: although they lack HLA-A and -B, they have at their surface a peculiar HLA protein that's almost never seen anywhere else in the body: HLA-G. The shape of HLA-G is very similar to the -A, -B, and -C proteins, but HLA-G differs from these other HLA proteins in that it doesn't vary much between each of us (it's one of the *non-classical* HLA proteins).[23]

The HLA-G gene was identified in the late 1980s, but it took many years to find out where it was used in the body.[24] Early evidence for the protein being used in the placenta sparked controversy – due to different views as to what constitutes proof of the presence of HLA-G. The problem is that there's such huge variability in HLA-A, -B and -C proteins that it is very difficult to get any reagent or process to reveal the presence of HLA-G specifically and not any other HLA protein.[25] Eventually, a consensus was reached that HLA-G is indeed on placen-tal trophoblast cells, and so the next question was: what does it do there?

Several of its features indicated that it would not do the same job as the other, more common, HLA proteins. For example, HLA-G stays at the surface of cells for a very long time, while other HLA proteins turn over to give an up-to-date report on what's being made inside each cell.[26] From 1995, attention focused on whether or not HLA-G on trophoblast cells would affect the NK cells that Bulmer, Moffett and Starkey had found to be abundant in the uterus during pregnancy. In 1996, several teams independently found that HLA-G was capable of *switching off* the killing action of NK cells.[27] The implication was that HLA-G on trophoblast cells marks these cells as special – specifically telling the mother's NK cells to leave these cells alone; these foetal cells are non-self but they are not dangerous. For such an important discovery, repetition of the experiment in different labs is needed to build confidence in the community, so it helped that different teams observed NK cells being switched off by HLA-G. But in fact, the teams disagreed over the way in which HLA-G did it. Researchers were at odds over how NK cells were able to detect the presence of HLA-G or, specifically, which receptors on NK cells could bind to HLA-G.

One possible cause of discrepancy was that each team was using their own lab's cells genetically altered to make HLA-G. To test whether or not this was a problem, one group requested a sample of the cells being used in another lab so that it could carry out a direct comparison. The request alone is enough to spark some feeling of ill trust, but things got far worse when the wrong cells were sent out. Somewhere along the line, one team's cells had been mixed up, so that, in fact, experiments thought to be done on cells having HLA-G had actually used cells genetically altered to make a different HLA protein instead. Not to name or shame any particular person or team, this anecdote shows how science progresses through everyday human errors, which in fact occur far more frequently than strokes of genius or even serendipitous breakthroughs.

In the end, it became clear that some of the data that had been published were plain wrong. No one's publications were ever formally retracted, or even officially corrected; just everyone in the community knew where the errors were. We know now that HLA-G can switch off immune cells in several ways, but it still remains unclear whether it affects all NK cells or only a fraction of them.[28] In any case, Moffett – and many others – think that the whole idea of it being critically important to switch off uterine NK cells has been one big red herring, a decade-long diversion because our thinking took a wrong turn.

As we've just discussed, it does seem to make sense that trophoblast cells – which lack normal HLA proteins – have the special HLA-G protein to switch off NK cells that would otherwise kill cells that are missing HLA proteins. Well, sort of – it still seems strange that so many NK cells are present in the uterus during pregnancy. They surely can't be there just to be turned off?

Moffett thinks that Medawar's question of how a mother's immune system gets switched off might have been the wrong thing to ask all along. Instead – Moffett thinks – we should be questioning why immune cells accumulate at the foetal–maternal interface in the first place. She's right; because a closer look at these uterine NK cells shows us that these cells aren't what they seemed at first.

NK cells from blood take their name – Natural Killers – for being good at killing diseased cells such as tumours, but it turns out that NK cells from the uterus are only weakly able to kill other cells. In fact, this was something Moffett reported early on but the observation was largely ignored for well over a decade. Everyone raced to work out how uterine NK cells were switched off without carefully considering whether or not they really need to be switched off.

Eventually, others caught up with Moffett. Several research teams – including Jack Strominger at Harvard, who had earlier worked with Bjorkman and Wiley to get the shape of the HLA protein – also found out that uterine NK cells were not good at killing.[29] In fact, Strominger established that the activity of hundreds of genes is different in uterine NK cells compared to blood NK cells.[30] The uterine cells get to keep the name 'Natural Killer' because they share many features with their blood counterparts – and they can deliver a lethal hit if pushed – but they don't seem to have a killer instinct. It may not be so important after all for trophoblast cells to use HLA-G as protection against NK cells in the uterus, because these immune cells can't kill very well anyway. And if killing isn't their thing, what do the NK cells in the placenta really do?

Yaqub (Jacob) Hanna, a Palestinian Arab working with Ofer

Mandelboim, an Israeli Jew, both at the Hebrew University in Jerusalem, discovered that NK cells – far from being involved in combat – actually secrete growth factors and other proteins which stimulate the invasion of trophoblast cells into the mother's uterus. The implication of this is that, far from killing other cells, NK cells in the uterus can help shape the structure of the placenta during early pregnancy.[31] Other researchers found that uterine NK cells also have a constructive role in mice (despite there being many differences between pregnancy in mice and that in people).[32] One study, for example, even found that a bone-marrow transplant – which provides an abundance of immune cells – can reverse certain reproductive problems in mice.[33] So, instead of being agents of destruction, NK cells in the uterus might actually aid blood flow in the placenta and help pregnancy succeed.[34]

This idea remains open to debate because it's very hard to test directly what NK cells really do inside a woman's uterus – and because uterine NK cells are hard to obtain in large numbers. Hanna and Mandelboim's study, for example, had to use tissue from more than 550 elective abortions.[35] To increase the numbers of uterine NK cells, scientists can culture them in the lab before beginning experiments. Some of the cell's properties could very well change when grown in the lab, and they may well behave differently from when they are in a uterus. But there is evidence that Hanna and Mandelboim's findings are relevant to NK cells in their natural environment.

Even though mouse anatomy is very different from human, mouse NK cells still interact with trophoblast cells in the uterus during pregnancy. And the activity of NK cells can influence how dilated the maternal uterine blood vessels become during pregnancy.[36] Mice don't get eclampsia or pre-eclampsia, but the level of blood supply in the uterus can directly affect their reproductive success in other ways. In mice, a high level of blood flow in the uterus can better support larger babies or an increased litter size. For that reason, many scientists think that NK cells help blood flow in a placenta; and that activating these immune cells is a benefit – not a hindrance – to pregnancy. So – even if anatomic details vary – there is evidence that pregnancy and immune-system genes are linked in many species.

If NK cells are there to help – and don't need to be switched off –

where does this leave HLA-G? What does this special HLA protein really do after all? Moffett, Mandelboim – and many others – simply say: we just don't know.[37] But the diversion of studying whether or not HLA-G can switch off NK cells has turned out to not be in vain. An ability of HLA-G to ward off immune cells, even to some extent, led research teams to discover that tumour cells – and perhaps other diseased cells – can usurp HLA-G for their own benefit. That is, some tumours make HLA-G themselves – to shield against an immune cell attack.[38] This indicates that HLA-G could, in fact, be a target for anti-tumour drugs – or perhaps used as a diagnostic marker for especially dangerous tumours.[39] Another potential medical use for HLA-G is that its ability to inhibit an immune response could be exploited to aid organ transplantation. Time will tell if these clinical applications prove viable.

All this information about trophoblast cells and NK cells in hand – fascinating as it is – doesn't answer Moffett's original question of why some women have pre-eclampsia and some don't. So, after Loke retired in 2002, Moffett decided that an altogether different approach was needed to directly test for the importance of our immune system in pregnancy. She decided to find out whether or not particular immune genes – or combinations of genes between each parent – make pregnancy more or less likely to be successful.

A specific idea about what to look for came to her in thinking through the details of how cells interact in the placenta: on the surface of trophoblast cells, there will be the baby's HLA-C proteins – which include those inherited from the father. These trophoblast cells contact the mother's uterine NK cells, and the HLA proteins they have could either weaken or strengthen the activity of the NK cells – depending on how the receptors on the mother's NK cells react to the versions of HLA-C inherited by the baby. This could influence the level of secretion of growth factors from the NK cells – which impacts blood flow in the placenta, in turn influencing whether or not pregnancy was successful. In this way, Moffett reasoned, the combination of the mother's NK cell receptor genes and the HLA-C genes inherited by the baby – including those from the father – could affect the success of pregnancy.

Family histories and population-based studies had already indicated that susceptibility to pre-eclampsia could be inherited, but nobody knew which genes were important. Moffett's idea was nice – but plenty of nice ideas fall by the wayside when tested rigorously. As Darwin's friend Thomas Huxley said: many a beautiful theory was killed by an ugly fact. To test her idea properly, Moffett had to set up a genetic study to find out if maternal NK cell genes and foetal HLA-C correlate with the success of pregnancy. To do this, genes were analysed in blood taken from 200 women with pre-eclampsia and a similar number of women who had normal pregnancies. Their babies' genes were analysed using umbilical-cord blood or mouth swabs.

Moffett found that no particular version of HLA-C on its own correlated to whether or not mothers had pre-eclampsia.[40] But the risk of pre-eclampsia was increased when certain versions of HLA-C genes were inherited by the baby *and* the mother had particular NK cell receptor genes. One way that these data can be interpreted is that certain combinations of genes between parents can lead to trophoblast cells switching off NK cells to some extent.[41] HLA-C is able to switch off NK cells – as we've discussed in the context of 'missing self'. So HLA proteins inherited by the baby could dampen activity of the mother's NK cells – depending on the specific versions of HLA-C inherited and which NK-cell receptor genes the mother has. This could lower the NK-cell secretion of growth factors, leading to insufficient blood flow in the placenta and in turn, problems in pregnancy. This is a plausible scenario – consistent with the genetic analysis of parents and babies – but in truth, it's not really known how these genes influence the frequency of pre-eclampsia. Even without understanding exactly how this works, these results show that differences in our immune-system genes can influence who gets born.

Defects in the placenta can cause other problems in pregnancy, not just pre-eclampsia – for example, recurrent miscarriage. Up to 3 per cent of couples in the UK have three or more consecutive miscarriages, which is more frequent than would be expected by chance – indicating that some couples are prone to miscarry. There are many issues that can underlie recurrent miscarriage, but one involves an insufficient blood flow in the placenta.[42] Moffett tested whether or not any particular combination of immune-system genes would be unusually frequent in couples who suffered recurrent miscarriages and discovered that – just like for pre-eclampsia – particular combinations of HLA-C *and* NK cell receptor genes correlated with the risk.[43] This time, her analysis revealed that a receptor protein that increases NK cell activity was protective.[44] This is, once again, consistent with the idea that activating uterine NK cells is good for pregnancy.

Moffett also found that poor growth of the baby – a condition formally called foetal growth restriction – similarly correlates with particular combinations of NK receptor genes and HLA-C.[45] The genetic link here again fits with the idea that activation of NK cells – and not too much inhibition – is important for a successful pregnancy. Altogether, Moffett's series of genetic studies indicate that pregnancy is wired to be more successful with couples having particular combinations of immune-system genes.

It's not that if you have this or that genetic inheritance you must have children with this or that other person, because these effects only slightly increase or decrease the relatively small risk of there being particular problems. As Isaac Asimov said, while thinking about the behaviour of gases: you can't tell what an individual molecule is going to do, but if you deal with trillions, quadrillions and quintillions, you can tell, very accurately, what they're going to do on the average.[46] Similarly here, these small effects don't predict who exactly will have problems in pregnancy – but they shape humanity overall.

We are only at the beginning of understanding this, but already there are many implications. First, there are potential medical benefits, as these discoveries seed new ideas for solving problems in fertility and pregnancy. Although it's not easy to predict which couples are likely to have a problem in pregnancy – because these immune-system genes only contribute a little to the overall risk – it could help to diagnose problems by checking the activity of uterine NK cells during pregnancy. The difficulty with this is in *how* to assess uterine NK cell activity. NK cells in blood taken from a mother's arm are obtained more easily than uterine NK cells, but it's not yet clear whether or not blood cells could report useful information that correlates to the state of cells in the uterus. It's also not clear – if a problem is detected – how best to manipulate the activity of NK cells in the uterus. Administration of hormones could alter the number of NK cells in the uterus, but we don't know yet whether or not the number of NK cells, rather than their state of activation, can influence pregnancy outcome.[47]

Upcoming clinical trials will assess the possibility of using drugs that manipulate NK cells to help with problems in pregnancy.[48]

Aside from seeding new ideas for medicine, these discoveries say something fundamental about human nature. It could just so happen that reproduction has co-opted use of these highly variable immune-system genes, and we shouldn't read into it any more than that, in the same way that it doesn't matter much that the *vas deferens* tube traffics sperm a longer way round than necessary. But to me, this is not like the *vas deferens* tube situation and it is almost certain that this does matter; that this genetic link between reproductive success and our ability to fight disease persists because it is beneficial.

There's not much cost to the *vas deferens* taking a detour on its way from the testicles to the urethra. So there's little pressure for the path this tube takes to be as short as possible. In contrast, there's an immense selective pressure on genes that influence the success of pregnancy or survival from disease, because these processes are so vitally close to what gets inherited; they determine directly who gets born and who lives. All other things being equal, genes that decrease the risk of a mother or baby dying at birth *must* propagate rapidly in the population.

This would be especially true historically – before medical interventions helped with difficult births. Sadly, even in the twenty-first century, around one in every hundred mothers dies in childbirth in countries where medical provision is poor.[49] This gives an estimate of the minimum frequency by which mothers die naturally during or shortly after childbirth. It indicates how strongly genes would be favoured if they could protect – even slightly – against maternal mortality, including those that protect against eclampsia.

Similarly, genes that can provide protection against infectious disease – especially against an illness which can be fatal before having children – must also propagate rapidly in the population (all else being equal). For as long as that disease was prevalent, such a gene or set of genes would rapidly increase in frequency in subsequent generations. Even protection against diseases that are not fatal can still impact the success of one's children and hence be selected for, through the generations. So variation in immune-system genes across all humanity is certain to be affected by their role in both reproduction *and* survival from disease.

This plays out as follows: some combinations of compatibility genes will be especially protective against a particular disease, and those versions propagate in the population. But successful pregnancy will have other requirements for variations of these very same genes. Versions of compatibility genes – and other immune-system genes – that favour successful reproduction will also be favoured in subsequent generations. These two pressures on the same sets of genes leads to a balance in what gets selected overall: a balance between versions of these genes that help us survive disease and those that help in pregnancy. In short, the outcome is to keep these genes diverse.

Despite this leap in understanding human nature, Medawar's paradox remains unsolved: we actually still don't fully understand how a baby is protected from the mother's immune system. But, by trying to find the answer, we know that uterine immune cells can help – not hinder – pregnancy. Many genes that regulate pregnancy and birth do not vary much between us. Yet the most variable of all our genes help construct this most intimate of contacts between people.

I suggest that this complex system is in place because no particular set of compatibility genes is perfect. The versions of compatibility genes you have inherited can make you more or less susceptible to various diseases, but there isn't a version of these genes that optimally protects for all possible diseases. This is likely why pregnancy – and interactions between cells in the placenta in particular – influences which versions of these genes get passed on to the next generation. In effect, the requirements for successful pregnancy help maintain our diversity in compatibility genes.

Without this process in place, one widespread lethal disease can favour particular versions of compatibility genes to be passed on, and cause our variation in these genes to narrow. This would make all of humanity especially susceptible to another disease – one not easily fought with the few compatibility genes left in the population. Admittedly, there's some fuzziness to how this works in detail, and more research needs to be done. Historians often call physics and mathematics the *exact* sciences, because biology is always a bit messier (at least for now).

The broad implication of all this is that the compatibility gene connects different aspects of our biology – from pregnancy to immunity – influencing how and when we die in a multitude of ways. Our diversity in these genes weaves a system for immune defence that works in each of us *and* across all of us. Six decades of exploration from Medawar to Moffett – and countless others in between – show the compatibility gene as our uniqueness *and* our togetherness.

Epilogue: What Makes You So Special?

The consequences of how our immune system works ripple out through much of human biology – a surprising amount of who and what we are has been influenced by our never-ceasing struggle to survive disease. It's the wonder of it all that's most important, and the reason why I wrote this book. But there's also the pragmatic issue of what our compatibility gene inheritance means to each of us in everyday life. Zoom in on a couple of particularly important examples – my wife and me. What diseases might we be more or less susceptible to? And, possibly even more important, according to the results from those smelly T-shirt experiments, just how compatible are we?

To find out, we each dribbled into small plastic tubes and sent them off for analysis. Before the answers came back, we had a couple of days to consider what the impact of the results might be. If our genes said that we are especially compatible, would that add to our relationship in any way? If the results come back that we are not ideally compatible, should I call a lawyer? Is love so blind that genes can be overlooked? Should we even find out about our compatibility genes, given that how long we have to live can be influenced by the versions we have? Our house became a waiting room. There was a sense that something intimate was about to be exposed.

Our spit arrived at Anthony Nolan – a UK charity that helps match transplantation donors and recipients. The tubes were bar-coded and shuffled down a series of robotic instruments that first isolated the DNA and then made copies of our compatibility genes. Small beads, each having a different short piece of DNA attached, are added to a solution containing our genes; beads with DNA just right to bind to one of our compatibility genes are picked out by a sensor, revealing which versions of these genes we have. This is how personal secrets are exposed in the twenty-first century.

So my wife, Katie, has the class I HLA genes A*02, A*03, B*07, B*27, Cw*01, Cw*07, and her class II genes are the variants classified as DRB1*01, DRB1*07, DRB4*01, DQA1*01, DQA1*02, DQB1*05 and DQB1*03. My own class I genes are those named A*30, A*68, B*44, B*13, Cw*06, Cw*05, while my class II genes are named DRB1*08, DRB1*11, DRB3*02, DQA1*04, DQA1*05, DQB1*03 and DQB1*04. A quick glance at the two lists by Steve Marsh – Deputy Director for Research at Anthony Nolan – reveals that I am very rare and my wife is rather common.

Immediately, it springs to mind that Wedekind's T-shirt experiment indicated that women prefer the scent of dissimilar versions of compatibility genes. By that reckoning – if my genes are exceptionally rare – everyone would find me sexually attractive. Well, that's a result I hadn't expected. Why didn't I know this when I was younger?

Trying to stay focused on the science – lost opportunities aside – I ask Marsh: just how rare am I? Marsh accesses an international database used for seeking transplant donors which lists the compatibility genes of 18 million people. Out of all these, there are just four like me. Four out of 18 million; I'm truly special (knew it). Even these four individuals – one in Germany and three in the US – may not be exactly like me. More precise analysis of the DNA would be done if we were really seeking a match for bone-marrow transplantation, because minor variations in compatibility genes weren't included in the analysis. After Marsh tells me these results, he looks at me and says plainly: just don't get ill. Any delusions of grandeur I had from thinking about my desirable scent are quashed by the realization that it's not going to be easy if I ever really do need to find a transplant donor.

When I say that my wife is common, sure her genes are more common than mine – but out of the 18 million in the database, there are only 185 people with genes like hers. Not quite the one in a million I always thought she was, but one in 100,000. Marsh himself has a particularly common set of compatibility genes, but even his only match a couple of hundred people out of the 18 million. The commonest set of HLA genes in the UK still only occurs with a frequency of less than 0.5 per cent. What makes you so special? Your immune system.

Looking at the issue in another way, nearly 6 per cent of people are without any match. That is, out of the 18 million people in the international database, over one million are *uniquely* defined by their compatibility genes. This puts the issue of sexual attractiveness in perspective. Aside from the controversy surrounding the experiments using smelly T-shirts and the like, even if it's true that women prefer the scent of men with compatibility genes dissimilar to their own, we're *all* pretty different.

Dating agencies that test HLA types to find your perfect soul-mate use computer algorithms which take into account the extent to which one version of a gene differs from another – that is, they don't just say A*02 is different from A*03, but they also assess how different these two variants are. But, overall, there's no evidence that this will help something as complex as a successful marriage. Genes are important – a carrot seed will never produce a turnip – but they are not the be all and end all. It's what you do with your genetic inheritance that counts. And my wife and I are compatible through shared experiences and magic.

As we discussed, there's a geographical structure to HLA types, and so the versions of compatibility genes we have also tell us about our ancestry. Since sets of compatibility genes are often inherited together, it can be established which of our genes are likely to have come together from each of our parents. For example, it is likely that I inherited A*68, B*44 and DRB1*08 from one parent and A*30, B*13 and DRB1*11 from the other parent, as these sets of genes are often found together in people. We can then examine where these sets of genes are usually found in the world.

My wife's HLA genes are found most frequently in Western Europe, consistent with her family being from that part of the world for as far back as we know. But something quite unexpected is the discovery that some of my wife's HLA genes are those that were found in Neanderthal DNA. Put simply, it is highly likely that my wife's ancestors bred with archaic humans. Nothing like that for me; I am so much more refined. And I look forward to discussing my wife's Neanderthal inheritance with her family at our next Christmas lunch.

For me, it turns out that one group of my HLA genes, A*30, B*13 and DRB1*11, are frequently found in Europe, particularly

Eastern Europe, while my other set, A*68, B*44 and DRB1*08, are common in India or Australia. This explains why my set of compatibility genes is so rare. It's not that any of the individual genes are unusual, but the combination of them is rare because they are usually found in different parts of the world. The Eastern European versions of my genes are likely to come from my maternal grandfather, who was born in Poland. And I have indeed been told that my natural father was born in India. I haven't seen my genetic father since I was a baby, because my parents divorced when I was very young. Before this moment, I had never considered that I have a genetic inheritance common in India. Something intimate has indeed been exposed.

Of course, these genes are best established as being important for our health. So what do our versions say about our own susceptibility or resistance to diseases? From the specific examples we've discussed, it is striking that my wife has inherited HLA-B*27; the version of HLA-B that would help if she ever suffered an infection with HIV but which also increases her susceptibility to the auto-immune disease ankylosing spondylitis. What does this mean practically? Nothing that's immediately life-changing, because the risk of ankylosing spondylitis is still extremely small. But if she ever develops back pain, the fact that she has HLA-B*27 would come to mind, and we might benefit from an early diagnosis should this auto-immune disease ever really develop.

Overall, nobody has a better or worse set of compatibility genes: there's no hierarchy in the system. The fact that we differ is what's important; the way our species has evolved to survive disease *requires* us to be different. This knowledge is, for me, the greatest gift that contemporary biology has given to society.

Bill Clinton, campaigning to be US president in 1992, emphasized how a country's finances underlie so much else: *It's the economy, stupid* was his catchphrase. If there's an analogous aspect of human physiology, a system of paramount importance which underpins a great deal of who and what we are, it's the immune system, stupid. *It's our overarching system.* We are each a fragment of a vast genetic tapestry forged from the way our species evolved to survive disease.

Notes

INTRODUCTION

1. Carrington, M. and Walker, B. D. Immunogenetics of spontaneous control of HIV. *Annual Review of Medicine* 63, 131–45 (2012).
2. Connor, S. Mystery of Aids immunity may be solved. *Independent* (5 November 2010).
3. The first dating agency offering this service began operating in the Boston area in 2007, as reported widely across the news media. See, for example: Nuzzo, R. Do I smell sexy? Here's a new reason to swap spit. *LA Times* (19 May 2008). However, the untimely death of the dating agency's founder and president Eric Holzle, in 2011, aged just forty-seven, leaves this particular company's future unclear.

CHAPTER 1: FRANKENSTEIN'S HOLY TRINITY

1. Medawar, P. B. *Memoir of a Thinking Radish* (Oxford University Press, 1986).
2. Medawar, J. *A Very Decided Preference: Life with Peter Medawar* (W. W. Norton and Company, 1990).
3. Mitchison, N. A. Interview online (2004). Interview of Av Mitchision by Martin Raff, June 2004, available online at 'Web of Stories': http://www.webofstories.com/play/13795?o=MS.
4. Nandy, D. *Sir Peter Medawar 1915–1987: A Personal Memoir* (Runnymede Trust, 1988).
5. Medawar, J. *A Very Decided Preference*.
6. Ibid.
7. Bhishagratna, K. K. L. *An English Translation of the Sushruta Samhita* (J. N. Bose, 1907).

8. Moore, A. Frankenstein's Cadillac. In *Dodgem Logic*, vol. 4, pp. 2–11 (Mad Love Publishing, 2010).

9. Jansson, S. Introduction to *Frankenstein by Mary Shelley, 1831 Edition* (Wordsworth Classics, 1999).

10. Gibson, T. and Medawar, P. B. The fate of skin homografts in man. *Journal of Anatomy* 77, 299–310, 294 (1943).

11. Medawar, P. B. The behaviour and fate of skin autografts and skin homografts in rabbits: a report to the War Wounds Committee of the Medical Research Council. *Journal of Anatomy* 78, 176–99 (1944).

12. Ibid., and Medawar, P. B. A second study of the behaviour and fate of skin homografts in rabbits: a report to the War Wounds Committee of the Medical Research Council. *Journal of Anatomy* 79, 157–76 (1945).

13. Medawar, P. B. *Memoir of a Thinking Radish*. Medawar, J. *A Very Decided Preference*.

14. Interview with Brigitte (Ita) Askonas, 29 May 2012.

15. Billingham, R. E., Brent, L. and Medawar, P. B. Actively acquired tolerance of foreign cells. *Nature* 172, 603–6 (1953).

16. Owen, R. D. Immunogenetic consequences of vascular anastomoses between bovine twins. *Science* 102, 400–401 (1945).

17. Brent, L. *Sunday's Child?* (Bank House Books, 2009).

18. E-mail correspondence with Leslie Brent, 1 June 2012.

19. Brent, L. Rupert Everett Billingham. 15 October 1921–16 November 2002: elected FRS 1961. *Biographical Memoirs of Fellows of the Royal Society* 51, 33–50 (2005).

20. Brent, L. *Sunday's Child?*

21. Ibid.

22. Ibid.

23. Ibid.

24. Ibid.

25. Ibid.

26. Brent. Rupert Everett Billingham.

27. Medawar, J. *A Very Decided Preference*.

28. Medawar, P. B. *Memoir of a Thinking Radish*.

29. Interview with Leslie Brent, 10 December 2010.

30. Brent. Rupert Everett Billingham.

31. Billingham, R. E., Brent, L. and Medawar, P. B. Quantitative studies on tissue transplantation immunity. iii. Actively acquired tolerance. *Philosophical Transactions of the Royal Society of London B Biological Sciences* 239, 357–414 (1956).

32. In a letter dated 24 October 1960 to Josh Lederburg, who had won the Nobel Prize for Medicine or Physiology two years earlier, Medawar wrote: 'Dear Joshua, I was absolutely delighted to get your telegram … I'm utterly delighted – with only the omissions of Ray Owen's and Billingham and Brent's names to make one regret the peremptory and arbitrary nature of these awards.'

33. Brent. *Sunday's Child?*

34. Letter from Medawar to Owen, 24 October 1960, reproduced in Hansen, P. J. Medawar redux – an overview on the use of farm animal models to elucidate principles of reproductive immunology. *American Journal of Reproductive Immunology* 64, 225–30 (2010).

35. Richard Dawkins spoke about two scientists that inspire him, Darwin and Medawar, at the National Portrait Gallery, London, 14 June 2012.

36. Medawar, P. B. The phenomenon of man. In *The Art of the Soluble*, 71–84 (Methuen and Co., 1967).

37. Klein, J. Interview for 'Web of Stories', http://www.webofstories.com/play/15857. (2005).

38. Klein, J. *Natural History of the Major Histocompatibility Complex* (John Wiley and Sons, 1986).

39. Medawar, P. B. Peter Alfred Gorer (1907–1961). *Biographical Memoirs of Fellows of the Royal Society* 7, 95–109 (1961).

40. Temple, R. Sir Peter Medawar. *New Scientist* 1405, 14–20 (1984).

41. Liz Simpson, as interviewed in the BBC TV *Horizon* documentary about Peter Medawar, broadcast in 1988.

42. Interview with Charles Medawar, 7 December 2010.

43. Ibid.

44. Stephen Jay Gould, Foreword to Medawar, P. B. *The Strange Case of the Spotted Mice* (Oxford University Press, 1996).

45. Interview with Liz Simpson, 3 December 2010.

46. Mitchison, N. A. Sir Peter Medawar (1915–1987). *Nature* 330, 112 (1987).

47. Interview with Av Mitchison, 30 March 2011. It is also of interest that Av's mother, Naomi, was a distinguished writer and James Watson's famous book *The Double Helix* is dedicated to her. Her brother was the famous Oxford geneticist J. B. S Haldane. Amongst other things, in 1933 J. B. S. Haldane postulated that transplant rejection was an immune reaction against alloantigens. Av's father was a Labour Member of Parliament.

48. A BBC TV documentary about Peter Medawar, in the series *Horizon*, broadcast in 1988.

49. Medawar, J. *A Very Decided Preference*.
50. Interview with Charles Medawar, 7 December 2010.
51. Brent. Rupert Everett Billingham.
52. E-mail correspondence with Leslie Brent, 1 June 2012.
53. Smith, L. Sale of human organs should be legalised, say surgeons. *Independent* (5 January 2011).

CHAPTER 2: SELF / NON-SELF

1. E-mail correspondence with Leslie Brent, March 2011.
2. Over the centuries, many great thinkers stamped their mark on defining the causes of disease even though, arguably, little changed fundamentally. The ninth-century CE Arab physician Rhazes, for example, through careful observations of patients, realized that smallpox and measles were different. Contemporary thinking was that smallpox was caused by a kind of fermentation that removed excess moisture from blood. Rhazes made the important observation that survivors of smallpox would rarely get the disease again, a hallmark of immunity. He interpreted this as being because all excess blood moisture had been removed during the first bout of illness, so that a second attack couldn't occur.
3. Horrox, R. *The Black Death* (Manchester University Press, 1994).
4. Silverstein, A. M. *A History of Immunology*, 2nd edn (Academic Press, 2009).
5. Debre, P. *Louis Pasteur* (The Johns Hopkins University Press, 2000).
6. Editorial. *Boston Medical and Surgical Journal* (1 March 1883).
7. *The Life Millennium* (Little, Brown and Company, 2000).
8. Burnet and Fenner were thinking specifically about how antibodies could be made. It was well established that in addition to white blood cells, our blood also contains soluble proteins called antibodies. These antibodies stick to and neutralize all kinds of germs and other potentially dangerous molecules. For Burnet and Fenner, and their contemporaries, the key problem lay in understanding how such antibodies could recognize so many different kinds of germs, while seemingly not triggering an attack on our own cells or tissue.
9. Fenner, F. *Nature, Nurture and Chance: The Lives of Frank and Charles Fenner* (Australian National University E Press, 2006).
10. Sweet, M. Obituary: Frank Fenner. *British Medical Journal* 341, 1218 (2010).
11. Interview with Elizabeth Dexter, MacFarlane Burnet's daughter, 9 February 2011.

12. Burnet, F. M. *Changing Patterns: An Atypical Biography* (Heinemann, 1968).

13. Interview with Elizabeth Dexter, 9 February 2011.

14. Sexton, C. *Burnet: A Life* (Oxford University Press, 1999).

15. Ibid.

16. Burnet, *Changing Patterns*.

17. Ibid.

18. Ibid.

19. Interview with Elizabeth Dexter, 9 February 2011.

20. Ibid.

21. Burnet. *Changing Patterns*.

22. Sexton. *Burnet: A Life*.

23. Interview with Elizabeth Dexter, 9 February 2011.

24. Owen, R. D. Immunogenetic consequences of vascular anastomoses between bovine twins. *Science* 102, 400–401 (1945).

25. Burnet, F. M. and Fenner, F. *The Production of Antibodies*, 2nd edn (Macmillan and Co., 1949).

26. Ibid.

27. Burnet. *Changing Patterns*.

28. Quoted in Soderqvist, T. *Science as Autobiography: The Troubled Life of Niels Jerne* (Yale University Press, 2003). This is a definitive and particularly thoughtful biography of Jerne. This biography uses a vast array of letters and interviews to paint a vivid picture of his life, with a great deal of interesting discussion and interpretion by the author.

29. Ibid.

30. Ibid.

31. Interview of Niels Jerne by Lewis Wolpert, recorded in 1987. It was not broadcast but is available from the online BBC archives. (The BBC archive states this was recorded in 1985, but the interview itself refers to 1987): http://www.bbc.co.uk/archive/scientists/10605.Shtml.

32. Ibid.

33. Ibid.

34. Ibid.

35. Ibid.

36. Burnet. *Changing Patterns*.

37. Burnet, F. M. A modification of Jerne's theory of antibody production using the concept of clonal selection. *The Australian Journal of Science* 20, 67–9 (1957).

38. Hodgkin, P. D., Heath, W. R. and Baxter, A. G. The clonal selection theory: 50 years since the revolution. *Nature Immunology* 8, 1019–26 (2007).

39. Burnet, F. M. A modification of Jerne's theory.

40. Burnet, F. M. *The Clonal Selection Theory of Acquired Immunity (The Abraham Flexner Lectures of Vanderbilt University 1958)* (Cambridge University Press, 1959).

41. Talmage, D. W. The acceptance and rejection of immunological concepts. *Annual Review of Immunology* 4, 1–11 (1986).

42. Hodgkin, Heath and Baxter. The clonal selection theory.

43. Talmage. The acceptance and rejection of immunological concepts.

44. Nossal, G. J. V. One cell – one antibody. In *Immunology: The Making of a Modern Science*, ed. Gallagher, R. B., Gilder, J., Nossal, G. J. V. and Salvatore, G. (Academic Press, 1995).

45. Nossal, G. J. Sir Gustav Nossal interviewed by Dr Max Blythe on 3 March 1987 and 1 April 1998. In *Interviews with Australian Scientists* (The Australian Academy of Scientists, 1998).

46. Nossal, G. J. and Lederberg, J. Antibody production by single cells. *Nature* 181, 1419–20 (1958).

47. Marchalonis, J. J. Burnet and Nossal: The impact on immunology of the Walter and Eliza Hall Institute. *The Quarterly Review of Biology* 69, 53–67 (1994).

48. Burnet, F. M. *Genes, Dreams and Realities* (Penguin Books, 1971). Burnet, F. M. *Endurance of Life* (Press Syndicate of the University of Cambridge, 1978).

49. Interview with Elizabeth Dexter, 9 February 2011.

50. Burnet. *Endurance of Life.*

51. Sexton. *Burnet: A Life.*

52. Talmage, D. W. Obituary: Frank Macfarlane Burnet 1899–1985. *Journal of Immunology* 136, 1528–9 (1986).

53. Brent, L. *A History of Transplantation Immunology* (Academic Press, 1997).

54. Miller, J. F. A. P. The discovery of thymus function. In *Immunology: The Making of a Modern Science*, ed. Gallagher et al.

55. Kincade, P. W. and Kelsoe, G. A birthday for B cells: Lymphopoiesis II, a scientific symposium honoring Max Cooper. *Nature Immunology* 4, 1155–7 (2003).

56. Or arguably over 150 years in the making, since Jenner first immunized a boy with smallpox.

57. Burnet. *Changing Patterns.*

58. Park, H. W. *Germs and Tissues: Frank Macfarlane Burnet, Peter Brian Medawar, and the Immunological Conjuncture* (Nova Science Publishers, 2010). This fifty-three-page monograph discusses in detail the approach of Burnet and Medawar.

CHAPTER 3: DEAD BUT ALIVE IN PARTS

1. Interview with Leslie Brent, 10 December 2010.
2. From James Watson in conversation with Brenda Maddox, 9 March 2011, London, organized by Intelligence Squared.
3. Brent, L. *A History of Transplantation Immunology* (Academic Press, 1997).
4. A definition of irreversible coma. Report of the Ad Hoc Committee of the Harvard Medical School to Examine the Definition of Brain Death. *JAMA* 205, 337–40 (1968).
5. The first succesful kidney transplant between living patients was performed in December 1954 at Brigham Hospital in Boston. This operation was performed between identical twins, which avoided the complication of an immune reaction effecting graft survival. For this and other work, the surgeon Joseph Murray won a Nobel Prize in 1990 along with Donnall Thomas, who developed bone-marrow transplantation as a cancer treatment.
6. Barnard, C. and Pepper, C. B. *One Life* (George G. Harrap and Co., 1969).
7. Ibid.
8. Ibid.
9. *Time* magazine. Cover story and feature article: Surgery: the ultimate operation. 15 December 1967.
10. Stark, T. *Knife to the Heart: The Story of Transplant Surgery* (Macmillan, 1996).
11. Congress. *Life-sustaining Technologies and the Elderly* (US Government Printing Office, 1987).
12. Rothman, D. J. *Strangers at the Bedside: A History of How Law and Bioethics Transformed Medical Decision Making* (Aldine de Gruyter, 2003).
13. Ibid.
14. Veatch, R. M. *Transplantation Ethics* (Georgetown University Press, 2000). This is a highly accessible and fascinating book that describes in far more detail than given here all the key issues around transplantation ethics, including more detailed views from different religious groups.
15. Caplan, A. L., Coelho D. H. (eds). *The Ethics of Organ Transplants* (Prometheus Books, 1998).
16. Numbers taken from the Mayo Clinic (US) and the National Health Service (UK), March 2011.

17. Speiser, P. and Smekal, F. G. *Karl Landsteiner*, trans. R. Rickett (Verlag Vienna, 1975).

18. Owen, R. Karl Landsteiner and the first human marker locus. *Genetics* 155, 995–8 (2000).

19. Gottlieb, A. M. Karl Landsteiner, the melancholy genius: his time and his colleagues, 1868–1943. *Transfusion Medicine Reviews* 12, 18–27 (1998). Karl Landsteiner's life was complex, and this is an interesting introduction.

20. Speiser, P. and Smekal, F. G. *Karl Landsteiner*.

21. Medawar, P. B. *The Uniqueness of the Individual* (Methuen and Co., 1957).

22. Rous, P. Karl Landsteiner. 1868–1943. *Obituary Notices of Fellows of the Royal Society* 5, 294–324 (1947).

23. Speiser, P. and Smekal, F. G. *Karl Landsteiner*.

24. In England, the relative frequency of the different blood groups are approximately 47 per cent O, 42 per cent A, 9 per cent B, and only 3 per cent AB.

25. Gottlieb. Karl Landsteiner, the melancholy genius.

26. Speiser and Smekal. *Karl Landsteiner*.

27. Henig, R. M. *A Monk and Two Peas: The Story of Gregor Mendel and the Discovery of Genetics* (Weidenfeld and Nicolson, 2000). This is a great, easy-to-read telling of Gregor Mendel's fascinating story.

28. Owen. Karl Landsteiner and the first human marker locus.

29. Beyond the A/B blood groups, the next most important issue in blood transfusions is the Rhesus factor. This was discovered in 1940 by US scientist Alexander Wiener, working with Landsteiner, who by that time had moved to New York's Rockefeller Institute to avoid the political troubles in Europe. The factor is named for the Rhesus monkey, whose cells were studied initially, and refers to a single type of protein that you either do or don't have on the surface of your red blood cells. Immune cells in someone who *doesn't* possess the Rhesus protein will react to blood cells from somebody who does – they would, in other words, recognize the protein as 'non-self'. There are many other differences between people that play a role in determining the success of blood transfusions, but the A/B blood groups and the Rhesus protein are the dominant factors.

30. Landsteiner, K. On individual differences in human blood. *Nobel Lectures, Physiology or Medicine* (1930).

31. Parham, P., Norman, P. J., Abi-Rached, L. and Guethlein, L. A. Human-specific evolution of killer cell immunoglobulin-like receptor recognition of major histocompatibility complex class I molecules. *Philosophical*

Transactions of the Royal Society of London B Biological Sciences 367, 800–811 (2012).

32. The fact that red blood cells lack compatibility proteins does make it hard for our body to detect anything dangerous that could live inside red blood cells, such as the malaria parasite.

33. In more detail, for a haematopoietic stem cell (bone-marrow) transplant it is hoped to be able to match 10/10 alleles across HLA-A, -B, -C, -DRB1 and -DQB1. For solid organ transplantation, HLA-A, -B, -C, -DRB1 and -DQB1 are assessed, but often some level of mismatch is unavoidable. In that case, much effort is spent on ensuring the recipient does not already have antibodies that could trigger a reaction against any of the HLA proteins on the donor's cells. Such antibodies could be present from exposure to other people's HLA proteins from pregnancy, blood transfusions or an earlier transplant.

34. Roberts, J. P. et al. Effect of changing the priority for HLA matching on the rates and outcomes of kidney transplantation in minority groups. *New England Journal of Medicine* 350, 545–51 (2004).

35. Thorsby, E. A short history of HLA. *Tissue Antigens* 74, 101–16 (2009). For more details on the history of HLA, this paper is a superb entry point, being exceptionally thorough and clear, with all the big papers cited within. Before these genes were discovered in humans they were first found in mice. Early clues came from Bernard Amos. Born in Kent and then working in Peter Gorer's laboratory in London, he showed that a mouse made antibodies against white blood cells from a different mouse strain, because of their different compatibility genes. This built on the pioneering work by Gorer and Snell that serologically defined the histocompatibility genes in mice, known as the H-2 system. Even though the mouse H-2 system was discovered before the HLA system, each came from parallel tracks of research using serology in each species. That is, HLA wasn't discovered through a direct search for the equivalent of H-2 in humans.

36. Dausset, J. The HLA adventure. In *History of HLA: Ten Recollections*, ed. Terasaki, P. L. (UCLA Tissue Typing Laboratory, 1990).

37. Van Rood, J. J. HLA and I. *Annual Review of Immunology* 11, 1–28 (1993).

38. Interview with Jon van Rood, 15 July 2011.

39. Dausset. The HLA adventure. Jan Klein recalls visiting Dausset's laboratory around 1958 and briefly discusses this on page 15 of his seminal book, *Natural History of the Major Histocompatibility Complex* (John Wiley and Sons, 1986).

40. Bodmer, W. and McKie, R. *The Book of Man* (Little, Brown and Company, 1994).

41. Interview with Sir Walter Bodmer, 25 May 2011.

42. Bodmer, J. and Bodmer, W. Rose Payne 1909–1999. With personal recollections by Julia and Walter Bodmer. *Tissue Antigens* 54, 102–5 (1999).

43. Dausset. The HLA adventure.

44. A brief history of the histocompatibility workshops is available online here: http://www.ihwg.org/about/history.Html.

45. At this meeting all fourteen groups used their improved techniques to test sera for reactivity against a common collection of cells isolated from forty-five different people.

46. Thorsby. A short history of HLA.

47. At the third HLA meeting, the teams tried to address the heredity of HLA by testing blood from eleven families, including some twins.

48. Thorsby. A short history of HLA.

49. Bodmer, W. F. HLA: what's in a name? A commentary on HLA nomenclature development over the years. *Tissue Antigens* 49, 293–6 (1997).

50. Walford, R. L. First meeting WHO Leukocyte Nomenclature Committee, New York, September, 1968. In *History of HLA: Ten Recollections*, ed. Terasaki.

51. Class I MHC proteins are also made from two chains, but one of them, given the unwieldy name of beta-2-microglobulin, does not vary from person to person.

52. The contemporary formal way of writing out HLA types and sub-types is to use an initial asterisk separator followed by subsequent fields separated with colons. As an example, one allele can be specified precisely as, say, HLA-A*02:101:01:02N. However, this level of detail is rarely used in scientific papers exploring the basic biology of HLA genes and proteins. It is more common to simply use a simple designation of say, HLA-A*02 or B*57, which strictly speaking covers a set of a few HLA types that have minor variations. Scientists will sometimes write a specific HLA type as say, HLA-B57 instead of its formal name of HLA-B*57. The HLA-C alleles include the designation w, to avoid confusion with other proteins called C1, C2, C3 and so on. Hence they are termed HLA-Cw*01, -Cw*02, -Cw*03, etc., and again, scientists will commonly omit the asterisk and talk of Cw1, Cw2 and so on. The HLA nomenclature also includes longer designations to fully account for subtle variations and up to four sets of numbers can follow the basic allele designation. Full information is available online, along with some description of the history in naming the HLA system, at: http://hla.alleles.org/nomenclature/naming.html.

53. Dausset. The HLA adventure.

54. Terasaki (ed.). *History of HLA: Ten Recollections.*
55. Two years prior to Dausset winning the Nobel Prize, van Rood won the Wolf Prize, a top prize awarded by Israel, along with Dausset and Snell. But for the Nobel Prize, his name was replaced by that of Baruch Benacerraf, who had earlier helped establish that there are genes that control immune responses, specifically the class II MHC genes.
56. Dausset. The HLA adventure.
57. Blueprints in the bloodstream. A BBC TV programme in the *Horizon* series, first broadcast in 1978.
58. Terasaki, P. L. History of HLA: a personalized view. In *History of HLA: Ten Recollections*, ed. Terasaki.
59. Hakim, N. S. and Papalois, V. E. (eds.). *History of Organ and Cell Transplantation* (Imperial College Press, 2003).
60. During the mid-1970s, some confusion arose because Terasaki's research indicated that HLA-matching was less important for deceased than for living donors. But later results across many studies clarified that HLA-matching was always beneficial in kidney transplantation.
61. Crispe, I. N. The liver as a lymphoid organ. *Annual Review of Immunology* 27, 147–63 (2009). This is a thorough review about the immunology in the liver by one of the world's experts in this subject.
62. Hornick, P. and Rose, R. (eds.). *Transplantation Immunology: Methods and Protocols* (Humana Press, 2010).
63. Laurance, J. Pig-to-human tissue transplants 'imminent'. *Independent* (21 October 2011).

CHAPTER 4: A CRYSTAL-CLEAR ANSWER AT LAST

1. Interview with Peter Doherty, 16 May 2011.
2. Butterfield, F. A Harvard Professor's baffling vanishing. *New York Times* (27 November 2001).
3. *Harvard University Gazette* (29 November 2001).
4. Who is a candidate for the Nobel Prize is generally a closely guarded secret. But people often do know, or assume, they are candidates through at least two routes. First, the Nobel Prize isn't the first prize somebody will win, and often it is clear someone is being considered if they have previously won other big international prizes. Second, gossip can fly around that reviews of a person's work are being solicited for their nomination and/or consideration by the relevant Nobel committee.
5. Feynman, R. There's plenty of room at the bottom. *Caltech Engineering and Science* 23, 22–36 (1960).

6. Watson, J. D. and Crick, F. H. C. Molecular structure of nucleic acids. *Nature* 171, 737–8 (1953).

7. E-mail correspondence with Pamela Bjorkman, 13 July 2012.

8. Schlesinger, S. Oral history: Don Wiley. Interviews with Don Wiley, recorded by Sondra Schlesinger 1 and 5 April 1999. Available at: http://virologyhistory. wustl. edu/wiley. Htm.

9. E-mail correspondence with Jack Strominger, 15 November 2011.

10. Discussion with Jim Kaufman, 27 May 2011.

11. E-mail correspondence with Jim Kaufman, Cambridge University, May 2011.

12. Strominger, J. L. The tortuous journey of a biochemist to immunoland and what he found there. *Annual Review of Immunology* 24, 1–31 (2006).

13. Interview with Jack Strominger, 13 June 2011.

14. Strominger. The tortuous journey.

15. E-mail correspondence with Jack Strominger, 15 November 2011.

16. Peter Parham had worked at getting the crystal structure of an HLA protein for a relatively brief time. He lost enthusiasm when a protein sample that took a month to obtain was very quickly lost when Wiley's lab took the sample for further purification. The anecdote emphasizes the essential quality that Pamela Bjorkman brought to the project: her dedication and hard work, which was needed to keep the project going over an incredibly long eight years. Getting a picture of HLA-A*02 was a long and arduous process. Parham remained enthusiastic about the work and discussed the project with Bjorkman often, especially at the time of writing up the paper when both were at Stanford University.

17. Interview with Pamela Bjorkman, 12 May 2011.

18. Beverley, P. and Naysmith, D. Obituary of Arnold Sanderson (1933–2011). *Immunology News: The Newsletter of the British Society for Immunology* 19.1, 10–12 (2012). Strominger's procedure for obtaining the HLA protein had involved many other researchers, most notably Arnold Sanderson. Sanderson had a colourful career and worked alongside many great immunologists. This obituary mentions that he thought that his own best work was on bacterial cell-wall sugars and that he enjoyed horse racing.

19. It later turned out that this cell line didn't actually have just one type of HLA-B. When sub-types were described afterwards so that each HLA allele could come in slightly different versions, the HLA-B*07 from this cell line turned out to include two different sub-types. This was described to me in e-mail correspondence with Jack Strominger, November 2011.

20. Discussion with Jim Kaufman, 27 May 2011.

21. Brewerton, D. *All About Arthritis: Past, Present, Future* (Harvard University Press, 1992). Chapter 20 of this book, entitled 'The beauty of crystals', contains a detailed discussion of the work by Bjorkman, Wiley and Strominger to get the crystal structure of HLA-A*02. The story is told from Bjorkman's perspective and includes a long letter written to the author by Bjorkman, describing many details of the process. This letter was written just a few years after the work was published, so details would be well remembered. This also serves to show how quickly this work was known to be important.

22. Interview with Pamela Bjorkman, 12 May 2011.

23. Rolf M. Zinkernagel – Autobiography. Available at Nobelprize. org.

24. A great deal of important research has been omitted here. Venezuelan immunologist Baruj Benacerraf, working at Harvard, had studied the genetic requirements for immune responses and discovered the so-called immune response (Ir) gene in guinea pigs. Independently, Hugh McDevitt, working in the UK's National Institute for Medical Research, London, showed that strains of mice would vary in their immune response. Benacerraff shared the 1980 Nobel Prize with Dausset and Snell. Snell shared the prize because his work with inbred strains of mice identified the genes that governed transplantation, which in turn made mice essential tools for probing the genetics of immune responses. Snell's work took a long time to be recognized: in 1956 when asked how many colleagues understood his work on compatibility genes, he replied that he could easily count them without using all his fingers. McDevitt must have been closely considered for the Nobel Prize in 1980 and many immunologists have said that he thoroughly deserved to win.

25. Interview with Rolf Zinkernagel, 18 May 2011.

26. Doherty, P. *The Beginner's Guide to Winning the Nobel Prize* (Columbia University Press, 2006).

27. Zinkernagel was experienced in doing this kind of experiment – to test how well cells are killed by immune cells. First, the cells that will be killed are filled with radioactivity. Then, as they get killed, their radioactive innards leak out into the surrounding liquid, indicating their death. Importantly, the number of cells killed is proportional to how radioactive the surrounding liquid gets.

28. Zinkernagel, R. M. Cellular immune recognition and the biological role of major transplantation antigens. Nobel lecture, 8 December 1996. This Nobel lecture gives a detailed and thorough account of Zinkernagel and Doherty's experiments and also outlines their influences at the time.

29. Zinkernagel, R. M. and Doherty, P. C. Restriction of in vitro T cell-mediated cytotoxicity in lymphocytic choriomeningitis within a syngeneic or semiallogeneic system. *Nature* 248, 701–2 (1974). Zinkernagel, R. M. and Doherty, P. C. Immunological surveillance against altered self components by sensitised T lymphocytes in lymphocytic choriomeningitis. *Nature* 251, 547–8 (1974).

30. Interview with Rolf Zinkernagel, 18 May 2011.

31. Interview with Peter Doherty, 16 May 2011.

32. Zinkernagel and Doherty. Restriction of in vitro T cell-mediated cytotoxicity.

33. Interview with Peter Doherty, 16 May 2011. Interview with Rolf Zinkernagel, 18 May 2011.

34. E-mail correspondence with Peter Doherty, 15 June 2011.

35. Doherty, P. C. and Zinkernagel, R. M. A biological role for the major histocompatibility antigens. *Lancet* 1, 1406–9 (1975).

36. Rebbeck, C. A., Thomas, R., Breen, M., Leroi, A. M. and Burt, A. Origins and evolution of a transmissible cancer. *Evolution* 63, 2340–49 (2009).

37. Interview with Peter Doherty, 16 May 2011.

38. Weiss, A. Discovering the TCR beta-chain by subtraction. *Journal of Immunology* 175, 2769–70 (2005). Much of the research behind the discovery of the T-cell receptor is not covered in depth in this book but is described succinctly in this brief overview by Art Weiss, where the key primary publications can be found also. Many great scientists played a role in the discovery of the T-cell receptor including Jim Allison, Ellis Reinherz, John Kappler and Philippa Marrack, who isolated antibodies that could detect the T-cell receptor. Mark Davis and Tak Mak's work led to identification of the relevant genes.

39. Hedrick, S. M., Cohen, D. I., Nielsen, E. A. and Davis, M. M. Isolation of cDNA clones encoding T cell-specific membrane-associated proteins. *Nature* 308, 149–53 (1984). Hedrick, S. M., Nielsen, E. A., Kavaler, J., Cohen, D. I. and Davis, M. M. Sequence relationships between putative T-cell receptor polypeptides and immunoglobulins. *Nature* 308, 153–8 (1984).

40. Discussion with Mark Davis, 2 November 2011.

41. Marx, J. L. Likely T cell receptor gene cloned. *Science* 221, 1278–9 (1983).

42. Hedrick, Cohen, Nielsen and Davis. Isolation of cDNA clones. Yanagi, Y. et al. A human T cell-specific cDNA clone encodes a protein having extensive homology to immunoglobulin chains. *Nature* 308, 145–9 (1984). Mark Davis had done his work with mouse cells and, independ-

ently, Tak Mak in Canada cloned a T-cell receptor gene from human cells.

43. Alain Townsend's PhD supervisor was Brigitte (Ita) Askonas, who had made many seminal contributions to immunology. A very large number of well-known immunologists trained with Askonas. Her obituary, by Bridget Ogilvie, is published in the *Guardian*, 10 January 2013.

44. Interview with Andrew McMichael, 4 July 2011.

45. Townsend, A. R., Gotch, F. M. and Davey, J. Cytotoxic T cells recognize fragments of the influenza nucleoprotein. *Cell* 42, 457–67 (1985).

46. Townsend, A. R. et al. The epitopes of influenza nucleoprotein recognized by cytotoxic T lymphocytes can be defined with short synthetic peptides. *Cell* 44, 959–68 (1986).

47. Interview with Alain Townsend, 25 May 2011.

48. Interview with Andrew McMichael, 4 July 2011.

49. Interview with Alain Townsend, 25 May 2011.

50. Galileo, G. *Sidereus Nuncius (or The Starry Messenger)* (1610). The original edition in New Latin is rare and worth hundreds of thousands of pounds. Various English translations are available, some free online.

51. E-mail correspondence with Peter Doherty, 15 June 2011.

52. In e-mail correspondence on 4 October 2011, Jack Strominger said that, while he didn't want to take anything away from Bjorkman and others, he 'never felt that Saper has gotten his fair share of credit for what turned out to be such an important paper'. Indeed Saper has missed out on the limelight for this work, compared with the others involved. He was second author of the original paper in *Nature* and was the first author of the longer, more detailed description of the structure of HLA-A*02 published later in 1991, while Strominger was on sabbatical leave in Oxford. The paper is: Saper, M. A., Bjorkman, P. J., and Wiley, D. C. Refined structure of the human histocompatibility antigen HLA-A2 at 2. 6 Å resolution. *Journal of Molecular Biology* 219, 277–319 (1991). Eminent immunologist Peter Parham called this second paper 'masterfully encyclopaedic'.

53. Bjorkman, P. J. Finding the groove. *Nature Immunology* 7, 787–9 (2006). In this article, Pamela Bjorkman details how the structure of HLA-A*02 was elucidated.

54. Parham, P. Putting a face to MHC restriction. *Journal of Immunology* 174, 3–5 (2005).

55. Braunstein, N. S. and Germain, R. N. Allele-specific control of Ia molecule surface expression and conformation: implications for a general model of Ia structure-function relationships. *Proceedings of the National*

Academy of Sciences USA 84, 2921–5 (1987). This paper, which slightly pre-dates the publication of the structure of the class I MHC protein HLA-A*02, did show a schematic view of how class II MHC protein would look, as predicted from many biochemical experiments. It got many essential features right, although of course the atomic-scale crystal structure of HLA-A*02 provided the definitive and iconic view.

56. Bjorkman, P. J. et al. Structure of the human class I histocompatibility antigen, HLA-A2. *Nature* 329, 506–12 (1987).

57. Bjorkman, P. J. et al. The foreign antigen binding site and T cell recognition regions of class I histocompatibility antigens. *Nature* 329, 512–18 (1987).

58. The valuable Canadian Gairdner award in 1994 included Wiley and Bjorkman but out left Strominger. Two years later, the Paul Ehrlich Prize, another major international award, included Bjorkman and Strominger and left out Wiley. Then, to complete all possible pairings, the Japan Prize, with its cash prize of around US $450,000, was given to Wiley and Strominger in 1999, leaving out Bjorkman. Scientists usually say in public that such prizes aren't overly important and certainly aren't anybody's focus, and it is true that the vast majority of successful scientists start with the drive and curiosity to find things out, not to become famous. On the other hand, there is considerable money and fame at stake with these international prizes, and a sprinkling of fairy dust from a Nobel can trigger global celebrity status (at least until the next one is awarded). Bjorkman, like many other scientists, says that prizes are great for highlighting discoveries widely but she also says there may be too many. Strominger suggests that recognition should be spread more widely because so much outstanding work is being done, in part because of the huge technical advances made in the past few decades. He thinks it might be better if each person could only win one big international award to spread the glory more widely. Zinkernagel says that the impact of prizes depends on one's character; for decent people, they won't change anything: 'They cause a problem only for people who are anyway intolerant.'

59. Doherty, P. *A Light History of Hot Air* (Melbourne University Press, 2008).

CHAPTER 5: DIFFERENCES BETWEEN US THAT MATTER

1. Guthrie's spirit lives on in the likes of singer-songwriter Billy Bragg in the UK and the band Wilco in the US, who teamed up in the late 1990s to record new songs using Guthrie's lyrics stored in archives kept by his

daughter Nora. Bragg says Guthrie was the greatest American lyrical poet of the twentieth century. Bragg, B. *Forward in Woody Guthrie: A Life* (Faber and Faber, 1999).

2. Nash, M. Memories of Woody Guthrie. *The New York Times* (9 February 2003).
3. Klein, J. *Woody Guthrie: A Life*, revised edn (Faber and Faber, 1999).
4. Ibid.
5. Ibid.
6. Dylan, B. *Chronicles: Volume One* (Simon and Schuster, 2004).
7. Details of the annual Woody Guthrie Folk Festival are at http://www.woodyguthrie.com.
8. MacDonald, M. E. A novel gene containing a trinucleotide repeat that is expanded and unstable on Huntington's disease chromosomes. The Huntington's Disease Collaborative Research Group. *Cell* 72, 971–83 (1993).
9. Walker, F. O. Huntington's disease. *Lancet* 369, 218–28 (2007).
10. Gordon Brown interviewed by Piers Morgan on *Piers Morgan's Life Stories*, first broadcast in the UK on 14 February 2010, ITV1.
11. Data from the World Health Organization, accessed June 2011: http://www.who.int/en.
12. Lilly, F., Boyse, E. A. and Old, L. J. Genetic basis of susceptibility to viral leukaemogenesis. *Lancet* 2, 1207–9 (1964). McDevitt, H. O. and Bodmer, W. F. HL-A, immune-response genes, and disease. *Lancet* 1, 1269–75 (1974).
13. Bodmer, W. and Bonilla, C. Common and rare variants in multifactorial susceptibility to common diseases. *Nature Genetics* 40, 695–701 (2008).
14. Bodmer, W. F. Genetic factors in Hodgkin's disease: association with a disease-susceptibility locus (DSA) in the HL-A region. *National Cancer Institute Monographs* 36, 127–34 (1973).
15. Schlosstein, L., Terasaki, P. I., Bluestone, R. and Pearson, C. M. High association of an HL-A antigen, W27, with ankylosing spondylitis. *New England Journal of Medicine* 288, 704–6 (1973).
16. Terasaki, P. I. History of HLA: a personalised view. In *History of HLA: Ten Recollections*, ed. Terasaki, P. I. (UCLA Tissue Typing Laboratory, 1990).
17. Brewerton, D. A. et al. Ankylosing spondylitis and HL-A 27. *Lancet* 1, 904–7 (1973).
18. Terasaki. History of HLA.
19. Brewerton, D. *All about Arthritis: Past, Present, Future* (Harvard University Press, 1995). Chapter 18 of this book, 'The race for answers',

describes Brewerton's view of how HLA became linked to disease, especially the work that linked HLA-B*27 to various diseases.

20. Interview with Derrick Brewerton, 5 July 2011.

21. Brewerton, D. A. Discovery: HLA and disease. *Current Opinion in Rheumatology* 15, 369–73 (2003). Brewerton gives here a personal account of his role in the early discoveries of the links between HLA and disease.

22. Ibid.

23. Interview with Derrick Brewerton, 5 July 2011.

24. Blueprints in the bloodstream. A BBC TV programme in the *Horizon* series, first broadcast in 1978.

25. Brewerton. *All about Arthritis.*

26. Brewerton. Discovery: HLA and disease.

27. Brewerton. *All about Arthritis*

28. Brewerton, D. *Felpham Beach* (Beach Publishers, 2011).

29. Interview with Derrick Brewerton, 5 July 2011.

30. Kaslow, R. A. et al. Influence of combinations of human major histocompatibility complex genes on the course of HIV-1 infection. *Nature Medicine* 2, 405–11 (1996).

31. Migueles, S. A. et al. HLA B*5701 is highly associated with restriction of virus replication in a subgroup of HIV-infected long term nonprogressors. *Proceedings of the National Academy of Sciences USA* 97, 2709–14 (2000).

32. Fellay, J. et al. A whole-genome association study of major determinants for host control of HIV-1. *Science* 317, 944–7 (2007).

33. Interview with Bruce Walker, 14 September 2011.

34. Lok, C. Vaccines: his best shot. *Nature* 473, 439–41 (2011).

35. Interview with Bruce Walker, 14 September 2011.

36. A variation on the often-quoted theme in Spider-Man comic books and movies, 'with great power comes great responsibility'.

37. Details of support from Mark and Lisa Schwartz are available in a press release from Mass General Hospital on 30 July 2008, entitled 'MGH receives $8.5 million grant from Schwartz Foundation to expand HIV/AIDS work in Africa', available here: http://www.massgeneral.org/about/pressrelease.aspx?id=1039. The Bill and Melinda Gates Foundation provides enormous resource and support for HIV research, and details are available at their web pages here: http://www.gatesfoundation.org/Pages/home.aspx.

38. Pereyra, F. et al. The major genetic determinants of HIV-1 control affect HLA class I peptide presentation. *Science* 330, 1551–7 (2010).

McMichael, A. J. and Jones, E. Y. Genetics. First-class control of HIV-1. *Science* 330, 1488–90 (2010).

39. Kaslow, R. A. et al. Influence of combinations of human major histocompatibility complex genes on the course of HIV-1 infection.

40. Migueles et al. HLA B*5701 is highly associated with restriction of virus replication in a subgroup of HIV-infected long-term non-progressors.

41. E-mail correspondence with Mary Carrington, 12 March 2012. To be precise, statistical significance depends on how many individuals are in the study – the CCR5 locus shows up if very large cohorts (n = thousands) are employed.

42. Bjorkman, P. J. et al. The foreign antigen binding site and T cell recognition regions of class I histocompatibility antigens. *Nature* 329, 512–18 (1987).

43. Interview with Andrew McMichael, 4 July 2011.

44. Evans, D. M. et al. Interaction between ERAP1 and HLA-B*27 in ankylosing spondylitis implicates peptide handling in the mechanism for HLA-B*27 in disease susceptibility. *Nature Genetics* (2011). This paper shows that the gene involved in directing peptides into HLA proteins was not associated with the rare form of ankylosing spondylitis in which patients don't have B*27. This is strong evidence that B*27 is involved in causing this auto-immune disease because of its role in presenting peptides to T cells. Allen, R. L., O'Callaghan, C. A., McMichael, A. J. and Bowness, P. Cutting edge: HLA-B*27 can form a novel beta 2-microglobulin-free heavy chain homodimer structure. *Journal of Immunology* 162, 5045–8 (1999). There are other possibilities to why B*27 causes this auto-immune disease. For example, this paper suggests that B*27 may adopt an unusual configuration in which two B*27 proteins stick together at cell surfaces. But this remains a controversial idea; another frontier of compatibility research.

45. Hill, A. V. et al. Molecular analysis of the association of HLA-B53 and resistance to severe malaria. *Nature* 360, 434–9 (1992).

CHAPTER 6: A PATH TO NEW MEDICINE

1. Interview with Rolf Zinkernagel, 18 May 2011.

2. Germain, R. Ron Germain: towards a grand unified theory. Interview by Amy Maxmen. *Journal of Experimental Medicine* 207, 266–7 (2010).

3. Genome-wide association studies: understanding the genetics of common disease. A symposium report published by the Academy of Medical Sciences, London, July 2009.

4. Schadt, E. E. Molecular networks as sensors and drivers of common human diseases. *Nature* 461, 218–23 (2009).

5. Friend, S. H. Something in common. *Science Translational Medicine* 2, 40ed46, http://stm.sciencemag.org (2010).

6. Interview with Eric Schadt, 23 August 2011.

7. Ibid.

8. Moukheiber, Z. Gene bully. *Forbes magazine* (9 July 2001). The article is available here: http://www.forbes.com/forbes/2001/0709/074.html.

9. Interview with Eric Schadt, 23 August 2011.

10. Ibid.

11. Suggested by Peter Parham in e-mail correspondence, 28 March 2012.

12. Medawar, P. B. *The Future of Man: The Reith Lectures 1959* (Methuen and Co., 1960).

13. Schadt, E. E., Linderman, M. D., Sorenson, J., Lee, L. and Nolan, G. P. Computational solutions to large-scale data management and analysis. *Nature Reviews Genetics* 11, 647–57 (2010).

14. Friend, S. H. Achievements of the past year. In *Sage Bionetworks*, available at: http://fora.tv/2011/04/15/Stephen_Friend_Achievements_of_the_Past_Year (2011).

15. This brief tale by Borges is widely available on the internet, in a translation by Andrew Hurley: https://notes. utk. edu/bio/greenberg. nsf/o/f2do3252 295eodo585256e120009adab?OpenDocument. Further tales are published in *Fictions* or the larger earlier collection entitled *Collected Fictions*, both published by Penguin. I'm grateful to Jorge Carneiro, head of the Theoretical Immunology Group at the Gulbenkian Institute of Science, Portugal, for bringing this work to my attention.

16. Chen, Y. et al. Variations in DNA elucidate molecular networks that cause disease. *Nature* 452, 429–35 (2008).

17. González, A. Merck will end Seattle research, costing 240 jobs. *Seattle Times* (23 October 2008).

18. Brown, D. Maker of Vioxx is accused of deception. *Washington Post* (16 April 2008).

19. Schadt et al. Computational solutions.

20. Kaiser, J. Profile: Stephen Friend. The visionary. *Science* 335, 651–3 (2012).

21. Sacks, J. *The Great Partnership: God, Science and the Search for Meaning* (Hodder and Stoughton, 2011).

22. Samson, M. et al. Resistance to HIV-1 infection in caucasian individuals bearing mutant alleles of the CCR-5 chemokine receptor gene. *Nature* 382, 722–5 (1996). Dean, M. et al. Genetic restriction of HIV-1 infec-

tion and progression to AIDS by a deletion allele of the CCR5 structural gene. *Science* 273, 1856–62 (1996).

23. Huang, Y. et al. The role of a mutant CCR5 allele in HIV-1 transmission and disease progression. *Nature Medicine* 2, 1240–43 (1996).

24. There is evidence that another factor is also able to protect haemophiliacs, but we still don't know what that factor is.

25. Hutter, G. et al. Long-term control of HIV by CCR5 Delta32/Delta32 stem-cell transplantation. *New England Journal of Medicine* 360, 692–8 (2009).

26. Hetherington, S. et al. Genetic variations in HLA-B region and hypersensitivity reactions to abacavir. *Lancet* 359, 1121–2 (2002). Mallal, S. et al. Association between presence of HLA-B*5701, HLA-DR*07, and HLA-DQ*03 and hypersensitivity to HIV-1 reverse-transcriptase inhibitor abacavir. *Lancet* 359, 727–32 (2002).

27. Mallal, S., et al. HLA-B*5701 screening for hypersensitivity to abacavir. *New England Journal of Medicine* 358, 568–79 (2008).

28. Facts taken from the Canadian AIDS Treatment Information Exchange, CATIE, http://www.catie.ca.

29. Chessman, D. et al. Human leukocyte antigen class I-restricted activation of CD8+ T cells provides the immunogenetic basis of a systemic drug hypersensitivity. *Immunity* 28, 822–32 (2008).

30. Another possibility would be that the drug somehow lowers the threshold at which T cells get activated so they react when they shouldn't – but if this is the case, it's not clear why the drug-triggered T cell response is restricted to people with a particular HLA type.

31. Chessman et al. Human leukocyte antigen class I-restricted activation of CD8+ T cells provides the immunogenetic basis of a systemic drug hypersensitivity

32. Oppenheimer, S. *Out of Eden: The Peopling of the World*, revised paperback edn (Robinson, 2004). This is one of many books that discuss this vast and fascinating subject.

33. Cann, R. L., Stoneking, M. and Wilson, A. C. Mitochondrial DNA and human evolution. *Nature* 325, 31–6 (1987).

34. Jakobsson, M. et al. Genotype, haplotype and copy-number variation in worldwide human populations. *Nature* 451, 998–1003 (2008). Li, J. Z. et al. Worldwide human relationships inferred from genome-wide patterns of variation. *Science* 319, 1100–1104 (2008). Sykes, B. *The Seven Daughters of Eve* (Bantam Press, 2001). The story of how our genes can be analysed to unravel our ancestry is lucidly told in this bestselling book.

35. Stix, G. Traces of a distant past. *Scientific American* 299, 56–63 (2008).

36. Abi-Rached, L. et al. The shaping of modern human immune systems by multiregional admixture with archaic humans. *Science* 334, 89–94 (2011).

37. Sanchez-Mazas, A. et al. Immunogenetics as a tool in anthropological studies. *Immunology* 133, 143–64 (2011). This paper includes many details about the relative frequencies of different HLA types across the world. Table 4 in this paper, for example, lists the four most frequent HLA types across ten different world regions.

38. Prugnolle, F. et al. Pathogen-driven selection and worldwide HLA class I diversity. *Current Biology* 15, 1022–7 (2005).

39. Belich, M. P. et al. Unusual HLA-B alleles in two tribes of Brazilian Indians. *Nature* 357, 326–9 (1992). Watkins, D. I. et al. New recombinant HLA-B alleles in a tribe of South American Amerindians indicate rapid evolution of MHC class I loci. *Nature* 357, 329–33 (1992).

40. Williams, R. C. and McAuley, J. E. HLA class I variation controlled for genetic admixture in the Gila River Indian community of Arizona: a model for the Paleo-Indians. *Human Immunology* 33, 39–46 (1992).

41. Sanchez-Mazas et al. Immunogenetics as a tool in anthropological studies.

42. This analysis was carried by the research group led by Professor Steven G. E. Marsh, Deputy Director of Research, Anthony Nolan Research Institute, Royal Free Hospital, London.

43. Poland, G. A., Ovsyannikova, I. G. and Jacobson, R. M. Genetics and immune responses to vaccines. In *Genetic Susceptibility to Infectious Diseases*, ed. Kaslow, R. A., McNicholl, J. M. and Hill, A. V. S. (Oxford University Press, 2008).

44. Cartron, G. et al. Therapeutic activity of humanized anti-CD20 monoclonal antibody and polymorphism in IgG Fc receptor FcgammaRIIIa gene. *Blood* 99, 754–8 (2002).

45. Chapman, M. A. et al. Initial genome sequencing and analysis of multiple myeloma. *Nature* 471, 467–72 (2011).

CHAPTER 7: MISSING SELF

1. E-mail correspondence from Rolf Kiessling, 5 September 2011.

2. Song lyric from 'Anthem', by Leonard Cohen, on the 1992 album *The Future* and the 2009 collection *Live in London*.

3. The use of animals in medical research is controversial for many of us. Throughout contemporary research in immunology, inbred mice have

facilitated many major advances, such as Zinkernagel and Doherty's Nobel-Prize-winning experiments that found a critical role for MHC proteins in the immunological detection of viruses. Today, hundreds of inbred strains of mice can be relatively easily purchased by appropriately licensed scientists. I am not advocating any particular view of this here other than the fact that it is absolutely right that the use of animals is always very carefully and critically questioned.

4. The phenomenon is known as 'hybrid resistance' because the F1 hybrid 'resists' bone-marrow transplants.

5. Cudkowicz, G. and Bennett, M. Peculiar immunobiology of bone marrow allografts. I. Graft rejection by irradiated responder mice. *Journal of Experimental Medicine* 134, 83–102 (1971).

6. Kiessling, R., Klein, E., Pross, H. and Wigzell, H. 'Natural' killer cells in the mouse. II. Cytotoxic cells with specificity for mouse Moloney leukemia cells. Characteristics of the killer cell. *European Journal of Immunology* 5, 117–21 (1975). Surprisingly, Kiessling published this landmark discovery in a relatively specialist European journal. When I asked about this in 2011, he said it was because he was fairly young and somewhat naive about the importance of maximizing exposure of one's work by trying to publish in the world's premiere journals. Herberman, R. B., Nunn, M. E. and Lavrin, D. H. Natural cytotoxic reactivity of mouse lymphoid cells against syngeneic acid allogeneic tumors. I. Distribution of reactivity and specificity. *International Journal of Cancer* 16, 216–29 (1975).

7. Kiessling and Herberman are the scientists celebrated for the discovery of the Natural Killer cell. However, this immune cell had been studied earlier in a different context from 1968 to 1970 by Ian MacLennan and colleagues at the University of Birmingham.

8. Interview with Rolf Kiessling, 7 September 2011.

9. E-mail correspondence from Rolf Kiessling, 10 September 2011.

10. Ibid.

11. Ibid.

12. Interview with Rolf Kiessling, 7 September 2011.

13. Herberman arrived in Pittsburgh when the new Cancer Institute had a staff of two but by the time he stepped down as its director, in 2009, it employed over 3,000.

14. Peterkin, T. US cancer expert Ronald Herberman warns against children using mobile phones. *Daily Telegraph* (24 July 2008).

15. Timonen, T., Saksela, E., Ranki, A. and Hayry, P. Fractionation, morphological and functional characterization of effector cells responsible for

human natural killer activity against cell-line targets. *Cellular Immunology* 48, 133–48 (1979).

16. Timonen, T., Ortaldo, J. R. and Herberman, R. B. Characteristics of human large granular lymphocytes and relationship to natural killer and K cells. *Journal of Experimental Medicine* 153, 569–82 (1981).

17. Kärre, K. How to recognize a foreign submarine. *Immunological Reviews* 155, 5–9 (1997).

18. Kärre, K. Natural killer cell recognition of missing self. *Nature Immunology* 9, 477–80 (2008).

19. Interview with Klas Kärre, 9 January, 2012.

20. Ibid.

21. Kärre. How to recognize a foreign submarine.

22. Cohen, G. B. et al. The selective downregulation of class I major histocompatibility complex proteins by HIV-1 protects HIV-infected cells from NK cells. *Immunity* 10, 661–71 (1999).

23. Interview with Klas Kärre, 9 January, 2012.

24. Lanier, L. L. Missing self, NK cells, and The White Album. *Journal of Immunology* 174, 6565 (2005).

25. Kärre, K., Ljunggren, H. G., Piontek, G. and Kiessling, R. Selective rejection of H-2-deficient lymphoma variants suggests alternative immune defence strategy. *Nature* 319, 675–8 (1986).

26. Ljunggren, H. G. and Kärre, K. In search of the 'missing self': MHC molecules and NK cell recognition. *Immunology Today* 11, 237–44 (1990).

27. Yokoyama, W. M. The search for the missing 'missing-self' receptor on natural killer cells. *Scandinavian Journal of Immunology* 55, 233–7 (2002).

28. Yokoyama, W. M., Jacobs, L. B., Kanagawa, O., Shevach, E. M. and Cohen, D. I. A murine T lymphocyte antigen belongs to a supergene family of type II integral membrane proteins. *Journal of Immunology* 143, 1379–86 (1989).

29. Yokoyama. The search for the missing 'missing-self' receptor on natural killer cells.

30. Interview with Wayne Yokoyama, 3 October 2011.

31. Ibid.

32. Ibid.

33. Over twenty years on from this basic discovery, my own research team uses super-resolving microscopes to visualize this killing machinery and to work out in detail how the inhibitory receptors regulate it. The hope is that, eventually, drugs can be designed to influence where and

when NK cells kill. Such drugs could be used in many medical treatments including helping target an attack on cancerous or virus-infected cells.

34. The Nobel Assembly at Karolinska Institutet awards the Nobel Prize in Physiology or Medicine. Nominations are evaluated by the Medical Nobel Committee, chaired by Klas Kärre in 2009 and 2010. Details can be accessed here: http://www.nobelprizemedicine.org/?page_id=326.

35. Colonna, M. and Samaridis, J. Cloning of immunoglobulin-superfamily members associated with HLA-C and HLA-B recognition by human natural killer cells. *Science* 268, 405–8 (1995). Wagtmann, N. et al. Molecular clones of the p58 NK cell receptor reveal immunoglobulin-related molecules with diversity in both the extra- and intracellular domains. *Immunity* 2, 439–49 (1995).

36. Scientists can not only add individual genes or proteins into mice, they can also include human cells. Hepatitis B and C viruses can't infect mouse liver cells as another example of the problem, but this could be solved by transplanting human liver into mice either directly or by using human stem cells in mice.

37. Khakoo, S. I. et al. HLA and NK cell inhibitory receptor genes in resolving hepatitis C virus infection. *Science* 305, 872–4 (2004).

38. Ge, D. et al. Genetic variation in IL28B predicts hepatitis C treatment-induced viral clearance. *Nature* 461, 399–401 (2009).

39. Khakoo et al. HLA and NK cell inhibitory receptor genes in resolving hepatitis C virus infection.

40. An alternative possibility is that the activating version of NK cell receptors might detect a specific viral peptide presented by an HLA protein, perhaps one from a common virus that we've evolved a specific defence against. Yet another possibility is that we make our own special peptide when under attack, and that gets recognized by an activating NK cell receptor to trigger an immune response. All in all, it's here that we hit an edge to our knowledge.

41. Bashirova, A. A., Thomas, R. and Carrington, M. HLA/KIR restraint of HIV: surviving the fittest. *Annual Review of Immunology* 29, 295–317 (2011).

42. Alter, G. et al. HIV-1 adaptation to NK-cell-mediated immune pressure. *Nature* 476, 96–100 (2011).

43. The modern overall view of NK cells is that they decide whether or not to kill another cell depending on the balance of signals received through their activating and inhibitory receptors, and Kärre's original hypothesis stands as one strategy this process facilitates.

CHAPTER 8: SEX AND SMELLY T-SHIRTS

1. Rimmel, E. *The Book of Perfumes* (Chapman and Hall, 1864). This book was a bestseller and was reprinted countless times. Various formats are readily available. Eugène Rimmel founded the brand 'Rimmel' with his father.

2. Turin, L. *The Secret of Scent: Adventures in Perfume and the Science of Smell* (Faber and Faber, 2006). Luca Turin advocates a specific view of how smell works. He suggests that how a molecule smells is determined by the frequencies at which different chemical bonds vibrate. His view is not widely accepted, in large part because there isn't a clear process that is established by which this information could be 'read' by our nose. A more conventional view is that shapes of different molecules are what is detected by our receptors for smell.

3. Luca Turin mentions his own analysis of this perfume in his TED talk, available online at: http://www.ted.com/talks/luca_turin_on_the_science_of_scent. html.

4. Turin. *The Secret of Scent.*

5. Medawar, P. B. *The Uniqueness of the Individual* (Basic Books, 1957).

6. Yamazaki, K. et al. Control of mating preferences in mice by genes in the major histocompatibility complex. *Journal of Experimental Medicine* 144, 1324–5 (1976).

7. Another member of their team, Tony Zayas, also noticed that mice had preferences for whom they mated with.

8. Thomas, L. *Lives of a Cell: Notes of a Biology Watcher* (Penguin, 1978).

9. Ibid.

10. Anonymous. Effects of sexual activity on beard growth in man. *Nature* 226, 869–70 (1970).

11. McClintock, M. K. Menstrual synchrony and suppression. *Nature* 229, 244–5 (1971).

12. Yang, Z. and Schank, J. C. Women do not synchronize their menstrual cycles. *Human Nature* 17, 434–47 (2006).

13. Beauchamp, G. K., Yamazaki, K. and Boyse, E. A. The chemosensory recognition of genetic individuality. *Scientific American* 253, 86–92 (1985).

14. Interview with Gary Beauchamp, 7 November 2011. Bard, J., Beauchamp, G. K. and Goldberg, E. H. Obituary: Edward A. Boyse. *Nature Immunology* 8, 1011–12 (2007).

15. Singh, P. B., Brown, R. E. and Roser, B. MHC antigens in urine as olfactory recognition cues. *Nature* 327, 161–4 (1987).

16. Manning, C. J., Wakeland, E. K. and Potts, W. K. Communal nesting patterns in mice implicate MHC genes in kin recognition. *Nature* 360, 581–3 (1992).

17. Potts, W. K., Manning, C. J. and Wakeland, E. K. Mating patterns in seminatural populations of mice influenced by MHC genotype. *Nature* 352, 619–21 (1991).

18. E-mail correspondence with Jon van Rood, 17 October 2011.

19. Wedekind, C., Seebeck, T., Bettens, F. and Paepke, A. J. MHC-dependent mate preferences in humans. *Proceedings: Biological Sciences* 260, 245–9 (1995).

20. Widmer, T. Der Schnüffeltest sticht unangenehm in die Nase (The sniffing test gets up people's noses). *Berner Zeitung* (1993).

21. E-mail correspondence with Claus Wedekind, 14 October 2011.

22. Interview with Claus Wedekind, 12 October 2011.

23. Reviews and correspondence between Wedekind and the journal *Nature* dating from 1 and 20 September 1994. Papers and original faxes passed on to me by Claus Wedekind, October 2011.

24. Interview with Claus Wedekind, 12 October 2011.

25. Letter from Professor William D. Hamilton, Department of Zoology, Oxford University, to Claus Wedekind, 6 December 1994. Hamilton died in 2000 and is often said to have been one of the world's leading evolutionary theorists of the twentieth century. Richard Dawkins, author of landmark books *The Selfish Gene* and *The God Delusion*, says that Hamilton was a great inspiration to him and has called him the greatest Darwinian since Darwin.

26. Ibid.

27. Richardson, S. Scent of a man. *Discover* magazine (February 1996). Available online here: http://discovermagazine.com/1996/feb/scentofaman699.

28. Interview with Claus Wedekind, 12 October 2011.

29. Testing a radical theory. *Nature Neuroscience* 7, 315 (2004). This sentiment has been attributed to James Randi in many places, although I'm not sure of its original source. Of relevance here, it was used in an editorial piece published in the top journal *Nature Neuroscience* when discussing data published in that journal which disagreed with Luca Turin's theory of smell.

30. Hedrick, P. and Loeschcke, V. MHC and mate selection in humans? *Trends in Ecology and Evolution* 11, 24 (1996).

31. Wedekind, C. and Seebeck, T. Reply from C. Wedekind and T. Seebeck. *Trends in Ecology and Evolution* 11, 24–5 (1996).

32. Interview with Claus Wedekind, 12 October 2011.

33. Roberts, S. C., Gosling, L. M., Carter, V. and Petrie, M. MHC-correlated odour preferences in humans and the use of oral contraceptives. *Proceedings: Biological Sciences* 275, 2715–22 (2008).

34. Jacob, S., McClintock, M. K., Zelano, B. and Ober, C. Paternally inherited HLA alleles are associated with women's choice of male odor. *Nature Genetics* 30, 175–9 (2002).

35. Potts, W. K. Wisdom through immunogenetics. *Nature Genetics* 30, 130–31 (2002).

36. Leinders-Zufall, T., Ishii, T., Mombaerts, P., Zufall, F. and Boehm, T. Structural requirements for the activation of vomeronasal sensory neurons by MHC peptides. *Nature Neuroscience* 12, 1551–8 (2009).

37. Kwak, J., Willse, A., Preti, G., Yamazaki, K. and Beauchamp, G. K. In search of the chemical basis for MHC odourtypes. *Proceedings: Biological Sciences* 277, 2417–25 (2010).

38. Interview with Gary Beauchamp, 7 November 2011.

39. Reusch, T. B., Haberli, M. A., Aeschlimann, P. B. and Milinski, M. Female sticklebacks count alleles in a strategy of sexual selection explaining MHC polymorphism. *Nature* 414, 300–302 (2001).

40. Ibid.

41. Kurtz, J. et al. Major histocompatibility complex diversity influences parasite resistance and innate immunity in sticklebacks. *Proceedings: Biological Science* 271, 197–204 (2004).

42. In fact, human smell is more sensitive than we commonly acknowledge and many scientists, including Gary Beauchamp for example, think we use olfaction far more than we generally realize.

43. Rosenberg, L. T., Cooperman, D. and Payne, R. HLA and mate selection. *Immunogenetics* 17, 89–93 (1983).

44. Havlicek, J. and Roberts, S. C. MHC-correlated mate choice in humans: a review. *Psychoneuroendocrinology* 34, 497–512 (2009).

45. Ober, C. et al. HLA and mate choice in humans. *American Journal of Human Genetics* 61, 497–504 (1997).

46. Interview with Gary Beauchamp, 7 November 2011.

CHAPTER 9: CONNECTIONS WITH THE MIND

1. Carla Shatz and her colleague Helen Blau discuss how they were hired and other interesting aspects of their career in a short film, *Pioneers of Science*, produced in 2010 by Stanford University, available here: http://www.youtube.com/watch?v=3tC1LneCuFs.

2. Gewin, V. Movers: Carla Shatz, director, BioX, Stanford University, Stanford, California. *Nature* 447, 610 (2007).

3. Interview with Carla Shatz, 23 November 2011.

4. http://www.youtube.com/watch?v=3tC1LneCuFs.

5. Interview with Carla Shatz, 23 November 2011.

6. Joly, E., Mucke, L. and Oldstone, M. B. Viral persistence in neurons explained by lack of major histocompatibility class I expression. *Science* 253, 1283–5 (1991).

7. Simpson, E. A historical perspective on immunological privilege. *Immunology Review* 213, 12–22 (2006).

8. Interview with Carla Shatz, 23 November 2011.

9. Ho, V. M., Lee, J. A. and Martin, K. C. The cell biology of synaptic plasticity. *Science* 334, 623–8 (2011).

10. How the brain works can't be studied without animal models, unfortunately. The key thing about the brain is the way in which the neural cells are connected to each other. So if isolated cells were studied, the essential nature of the brain would be lost. Cats have been especially important in studying synaptic circuits involved in vision, because they have eyes facing the front, use binocular vision, and the layout of their visual system is similar to ours. Undoubtedly, scientists carry out this kind of research in the most humane way possible, with animals being anesthetized, for example, and as few animals as possible being used.

11. Hubel, D. and Wiesel, T. *Brain and Visual Perception: The Story of a 25-year Collaboration* (Oxford University Press, 2005).

12. A fascinating insight into this work is discussed in David Hubel's Nobel Lecture, given on 8 December 1981 at the Karolinska Institute, which can be viewed at: http://www.nobelprize.org/mediaplayer/index.php?id=1605andview=1.

13. Hubel and Wiesel. *Brain and Visual Perception*.

14. Ibid.

15. Olby, R. *Francis Crick: Hunter of Life's Secrets* (Cold Spring Harbor Laboratory Press, 2008).

16. Hubel and Wiesel. *Brain and Visual Perception*.

17. In a more holistic sense, consciousness is obviously what sets aside a brain from a computer, but we have little idea how that works or even what it is: it's the biggest unknown.

18. Corriveau, R. A., Huh, G. S. and Shatz, C. J. Regulation of class I MHC gene expression in the developing and mature CNS by neural activity. *Neuron* 21, 505–20 (1998).

19. Interview with Carla Shatz, 23 November 2011.

20. Huh, G. S. et al. Functional requirement for class I MHC in CNS development and plasticity. *Science* 290, 2155–9 (2000).

21. Marcus, A. and Oransky, I. Science publishing: the paper is not sacred. *Nature* 480, 449–50 (2011).

22. Purcell, S. M. et al. Common polygenic variation contributes to risk of schizophrenia and bipolar disorder. *Nature* 460, 748–52 (2009). Stefansson, H. et al. Common variants conferring risk of schizophrenia. *Nature* 460, 744–7 (2009).

23. Wright, P., Nimgaonkar, V., R. G. and Murray, R. M. HLA and psychiatric disease. In *HLA in Health and Disease*, ed. Lechler, R. and Warrens, A. (Academic Press, 2000).

24. Numbers are taken from from Narcolepsy UK, where far more information is also available: http://www.narcolepsy.org.uk/.

25. Hor, H. et al. Genome-wide association study identifies new HLA class II haplotypes strongly protective against narcolepsy. *Nature Genetics* 42, 786–9 (2010).

26. Cvetkovic-Lopes, V. et al. Elevated Tribbles homolog 2-specific antibody levels in narcolepsy patients. *Journal of Clinical Investigation* 120, 713–19 (2010).

27. Boulanger, L. M. and Shatz, C. J. Immune signalling in neural development, synaptic plasticity and disease. *Nature Reviews Neuroscience* 5, 521–31 (2004).

28. McConnell, M. J., Huang, Y. H., Datwani, A. and Shatz, C. J. H2-K(b) and H2-D(b) regulate cerebellar long-term depression and limit motor learning. *Proceedings of the National Academy of Sciences USA* 106, 6784–9 (2009).

29. Neuroscience 2011, Washington, DC, 12–16 November 2011: http://www.sfn.org/am2011/home. aspx.

30. Abstracts from all the presentations of this meeting are available online through the Society for Neuroscience and many tens of these abstracts discuss immune-system genes or proteins in various aspects of brain research.

31. Tang, S. C. et al. Pivotal role for neuronal Toll-like receptors in ischemic brain injury and functional deficits. *Proceedings of the National Academy of Sciences USA* 104, 13798–803 (2007).

32. Allan, S. M., Tyrrell, P. J. and Rothwell, N. J. Interleukin-1 and neuronal injury. *Nature Reviews Immunology* 5, 629–40 (2005).

33. Interview with Carla Shatz, 23 November 2011.

34. Irwin, M. R. and Cole, S. W. Reciprocal regulation of the neural and innate immune systems. *Nature Reviews Immunology* 11, 625–32 (2011).

35. Gleeson, M. et al. The anti-inflammatory effects of exercise: mechanisms and implications for the prevention and treatment of disease. *Nature Reviews Immunology* 11, 607–15 (2011).

36. Paul, W. E. and Seder, R. A. Lymphocyte responses and cytokines. *Cell* 76, 241–51 (1994). This paper was influential for scientists thinking about the similarities in how immune cells and neurons work. Mike Norcross, then working with Ron Germain at the National Institute of Health, had earlier suggested the terminology of an 'immune synapse' to decsribe the contact a T cell makes with other cells, but the paper by Paul and Seder reached a much wider audience.

37. Poo, W. J., Conrad, L. and Janeway, C. A., Jr. Receptor-directed focusing of lymphokine release by helper T cells. *Nature* 332, 378–80 (1988).

38. Monks, C. R., Freiberg, B. A., Kupfer, H., Sciaky, N. and Kupfer, A. Three-dimensional segregation of supramolecular activation clusters in T cells. *Nature* 395, 82–6 (1998).

39. Davis, D. M. Intrigue at the immune synapse. *Scientific American* 294, 48–55 (2006). My discussion of Avi Kupfer's research in this book is similar to my article about his work, published in *Scientific American*.

40. E-mail correspondence with Anton van der Merwe, 15 November 2004.

41. Grakoui, A. et al. The immunological synapse: a molecular machine controlling T cell activation. *Science* 285, 221–7 (1999).

42. Davis, D. M. et al. The human natural killer cell immune synapse. *Proceedings of the National Academy of Sciences USA* 96, 15062–7 (1999).

43. Davis, D. M. and Sowinski, S. Membrane nanotubes: dynamic long-distance connections between animal cells. *Nature Reviews Molecular Cell Biology* 9, 431–6 (2008).

44. Sowinski, S. et al. Membrane nanotubes physically connect T cells over long distances presenting a novel route for HIV-1 transmission. *Nature Cell Biology* 10, 211–19 (2008).

45. Gousset, K. et al. Prions hijack tunnelling nanotubes for intercellular spread. *Nature Cell Biology* 11, 328–36 (2009).

46. Kwok, R. Cell biology: the new cell anatomy. *Nature* 480, 26–8 (2011).

47. Hubel, D. *Eye, Brain and Vision* (Scientific American Library, 1988).

CHAPTER 10: COMPATIBILITY FOR SUCCESSFUL PREGNANCY

1. Billington, W. D. The immunological problem of pregnancy: 50 years with the hope of progress. A tribute to Peter Medawar. *Journal of Reproductive Immunology* 60, 1–11 (2003). Medawar, P. B. Some immunological

and endocrinological problems raised by the evolution of viviparity in vertebrates. *Symposia of the Society for Experimental Biology* 7, 320–38 (1953).

2. Medawar, P. B. Some immunological and endocrinological problems.

3. Moffett-King, A. Natural killer cells and pregnancy. *Nature Reviews Immunology* 2, 656–63 (2002).

4. Ibid.

5. Billingham, R. E. Transplantation immunity and the maternal-fetal relation (part one). *New England Journal of Medicine* 270, 667–72 (1964). Billingham, R. E. Transplantation immunity and the maternal–fetal relation (continued: part 2). *New England Journal of Medicine* 270, 720–25 (1964).

6. Apps, R. et al. Human leucocyte antigen (HLA) expression of primary trophoblast cells and placental cell lines, determined using single antigen beads to characterize allotype specificities of anti-HLA antibodies. *Immunology* 127, 26–39 (2009).

7. An hour-long interview with Charlie Loke filmed by Alan Macfarlane on 22 February 2007 is available in archives held at the University of Cambridge. In this wide-ranging interview, Loke discusses his background, personal life and some of his work in the immunology of pregnancy. The full interview is available online: http://www.dspace.cam.ac.uk/handle/1810/194470.

8. Moffett, A. Charlie Loke: contributions from Tennis Court Road – past, present and future. *Placenta* 24 Suppl. A, S4-9 (2003).

9. http://www.dspace.cam.ac.uk/handle/1810/194470.

10. Moffett. Charlie Loke.

11. Interview with Ashley Moffett, 19 January 2012.

12. Moffett. Charlie Loke.

13. Interview with Ashley Moffett, 19 January 2012.

14. Ashley Moffett's work at this time uses her married name, King. After divorce, she used Moffett-King for a few publications and then later her maiden name, Moffett. At the time she was going through her divorce, she was particularly worried about being able to carry on with her top-level research career while raising three children as a single mother. At a dinner, she happened to sit across from a very famous female scientist who she knew also had children and was divorced. So she asked her how she coped, and the woman replied very clearly: 'Come on, Ashley, of course it's much easier to deal with three children compared with having to cope with three children *and* a husband.'

15. Interview with Ashley Moffett, 19 January 2012.

16. Ibid.
17. Ibid.
18. King, A., Wellings, V., Gardner, L. and Loke, Y. W. Immunocytochemical characterization of the unusual large granular lymphocytes in human endometrium throughout the menstrual cycle. *Human Immunology* 24, 195–205 (1989).
19. Interview with Ashley Moffett, 19 January 2012.
20. Bulmer, J. N., Morrison, L., Longfellow, M., Ritson, A. and Pace, D. Granulated lymphocytes in human endometrium: histochemical and immunohistochemical studies. *Human Reproduction* 6, 791–8 (1991). Starkey, P. M., Sargent, I. L. and Redman, C. W. Cell populations in human early pregnancy decidua: characterization and isolation of large granular lymphocytes by flow cytometry. *Immunology* 65, 129–34 (1988).
21. Interview with Phyllis Starkey MP by Richard Reece, published in the *Biochemist* magazine, June 2006, available here: http://www.biochemist. org/bio/02803/0049/028030049.pdf.
22. Interview with Ashley Moffett, 19 January 2012.
23. Clements, C. S. et al. Crystal structure of HLA-G: a non-classical MHC class I molecule expressed at the fetal–maternal interface. *Proceedings of the National Academy of Sciences USA* 102, 3360–65 (2005).
24. Geraghty, D. E., Koller, B. H. and Orr, H. T. A human major histocompatibility complex class I gene that encodes a protein with a shortened cytoplasmic segment. *Proceedings of the National Academy of Sciences USA* 84, 9145–9 (1987). Kovats, S. et al. A class I antigen, HLA-G, expressed in human trophoblasts. *Science* 248, 220–23 (1990). Ellis, S. A., Palmer, M. S. and McMichael, A. J. Human trophoblast and the choriocarcinoma cell line BeWo express a truncated HLA Class I molecule. *Journal of Immunology* 144, 731–5 (1990).
25. Apps, R., Gardner, L. and Moffett, A. A critical look at HLA-G. *Trends in Immunology* 29, 313–21 (2008).
26. Davis, D. M. et al. Impaired spontaneous endocytosis of HLA-G. *European Journal of Immunology* 27, 2714–19 (1997).
27. Rouas-Freiss, N., Goncalves, R. M., Menier, C., Dausset, J. and Carosella, E. D. Direct evidence to support the role of HLA-G in protecting the fetus from maternal uterine natural killer cytolysis. *Proceedings of the National Academy of Sciences USA* 94, 11520–25 (1997). Pazmany, L. et al. Protection from natural killer cell-mediated lysis by HLA-G expression on target cells. *Science* 274, 792–5 (1996). Soderstrom, K., Corliss, B., Lanier, L. L. and Phillips, J. H. CD94/NKG2 is the

predominant inhibitory receptor involved in recognition of HLA-G by decidual and peripheral blood NK cells. *Journal of Immunology* 159, 1072–5 (1997). Ponte, M. et al. Inhibitory receptors sensing HLA-G1 molecules in pregnancy: decidua-associated natural killer cells express LIR-1 and CD94/NKG2A and acquire p49, an HLA-G1-specific receptor. *Proceedings of the National Academy of Sciences USA* 96, 5674–9 (1999).

28. In detail, HLA-G can also work indirectly, through HLA-E. Expression of HLA-G allows HLA-E to get to the cell surface and HLA-E can then also be involved in inhibiting NK cells from killing trophoblast cells.

29. Kopcow, H. D. et al. Human decidual NK cells form immature activating synapses and are not cytotoxic. *Proceedings of the National Academy of Sciences USA* 102, 15563–8 (2005).

30. Koopman, L. A. et al. Human decidual natural killer cells are a unique NK cell subset with immunomodulatory potential. *Journal of Experimental Medicine* 198, 1201–12 (2003).

31. Hanna, J. et al. Decidual NK cells regulate key developmental processes at the human fetal–maternal interface. *Nature Medicine* 12, 1065–74 (2006).

32. Croy, B. A. et al. Uterine natural killer cells: insights into their cellular and molecular biology from mouse modelling. *Reproduction* 126, 149–60 (2003).

33. Guimond, M. J., Wang, B. and Croy, B. A. Engraftment of bone marrow from severe combined immunodeficient (SCID) mice reverses the reproductive deficits in natural killer cell-deficient tg epsilon 26 mice. *Journal of Experimental Medicine* 187, 217–23 (1998).

34. Hanna, J. and Mandelboim, O. When killers become helpers. *Trends in Immunology* 28, 201–6 (2007).

35. Koopman et al. Human decidual natural killer cells.

36. Madeja, Z. et al. Paternal MHC expression on mouse trophoblast affects uterine vascularization and fetal growth. *Proceedings of the National Academy of Sciences USA* 108, 4012–17 (2011).

37. Interview with Ashley Moffett, 19 January 2012. E-mail correspondence with Ofer Mandelboim, 24 January 2012.

38. Carosella, E. D., Moreau, P., Lemaoult, J. and Rouas-Freiss, N. HLA-G: from biology to clinical benefits. *Trends in immunology* 29, 125–32 (2008). Paul, P., et al. HLA-G expression in melanoma: a way for tumor cells to escape from immunosurveillance. *Proceedings of the National Academy of Sciences USA* 95, 4510–15 (1998).

39. Carosella, E. D., Favier, B., Rouas-Freiss, N., Moreau, P. and Lemaoult, J. Beyond the increasing complexity of the immunomodulatory HLA-G molecule. *Blood* 111, 4862–70 (2008).

40. Hiby, S. E. et al. Combinations of maternal KIR and fetal HLA-C genes influence the risk of preeclampsia and reproductive success. *Journal of Experimental Medicine* 200, 957–65 (2004).

41. Ibid.

42. Further details on recurrent miscarriage are available from the Royal College of Obstetricians and Gynaecologists in London, UK, here: http://www.rcog.org.uk/womens-health/clinical-guidance/couples-recurrent-miscarriage-what-rcog-guideline-means-you.

43. Hiby, S. E. et al. Association of maternal killer-cell immunoglobulin-like receptors and parental HLA-C genotypes with recurrent miscarriage. *Human Reproduction* 23, 972–6 (2008).

44. Ibid.

45. Hiby, S. E. et al. Maternal activating KIRs protect against human reproductive failure mediated by fetal HLA-C2. *Journal of Clinical Investigation* 120, 4102–10 (2010).

46. Taken from an interview with Isaac Asimov in 1990, available on the CD *Science Fiction Writers*, published by the British Library, 2011.

47. Tang, A. W., Alfirevic, Z. and Quenby, S. Natural killer cells and pregnancy outcomes in women with recurrent miscarriage and infertility: a systematic review. *Human Reproduction* 26, 1971–80 (2011).

48. Tang, A. W. and Quenby, S. Recent thoughts on management and prevention of recurrent early pregnancy loss. *Current Opinion in Obstetrics and Gynecology* 22, 446–51 (2010).

49. Hogan, M. C. et al. Maternal mortality for 181 countries, 1980–2008: a systematic analysis of progress towards Millennium Development Goal 5. *Lancet* 375, 1609–23 (2010).

Index